OLD DOGS
NEW TRICKS

OLD DOGS NEW TRICKS

MORE TALES FROM TWO KIWI COUNTRY VETS

Peter Jerram & Peter Anderson
Authors of *Cock and Bull Stories*

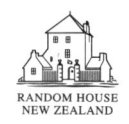

RANDOM HOUSE

UK | USA | Canada | Ireland | Australia
India | New Zealand | South Africa | China

Random House is an imprint of the Penguin Random House group of companies, whose addresses can be found at global.penguinrandomhouse.com.

Penguin
Random House
New Zealand

First published by Penguin Random House New Zealand, 2016

10 9 8 7 6 5 4 3 2 1

Text © Peter Jerram and Peter Anderson, 2016

The moral right of the authors has been asserted.

All rights reserved. Without limiting the rights under copyright reserved above, no part of this publication may be reproduced, stored in or introduced into a retrieval system, or transmitted, in any form or by any means (electronic, mechanical, photocopying, recording or otherwise), without the prior written permission of both the copyright owner and the above publisher of this book.

Cover design by Carla Sy © Penguin Random House New Zealand
Internal design by Megan van Staden
Typesetting by Carla Sy
Cover and internal illustrations by Ashley Smith

Printed and bound in Australia by Griffin Press, an Accredited ISO AS/NZS 14001 Environmental Management Systems Printer

A catalogue record for this book is available from the National Library of New Zealand.

ISBN 978-1-77553-886-8
eISBN 978-1-77553-887-5

www.penguin.co.nz

MIX
Paper from responsible sources
FSC® C009448

For our wonderful and remarkable children: Caroline, Tom, George, Jane and Pippa. You've been a huge part of all this, and we hope the book will give you some insight into what your missing fathers were doing.

CONTENTS

Foreword	9
Why Do We Do It? — PJ	13
My Reasons — PA	16
A True Gentleman — PJ	19
Predictably Unpredictable — PA	23
At the Bluff — PJ	31
Just Do It — PA	41
Angora Anguish — PJ	47
Hoof to Propeller — PA	59
Don't Bite the Hand — PJ	65
A Long Day on D'Urville — PA	73
Wacker — PJ	81
Drug Shrinkage — PA	87
Consummate Professionals — PJ	93
The Muller — PJ	99
The Lord God Made Them All — PA	105
The Bench Class — PJ	113
Damage and Dung — PA	119
Admiral Jerram — PJ	127

To Catch a Thief — PA	**131**
A Hard Man — PJ	**137**
Tooted Pachyderms — PA	**143**
Life or Death — PJ	**159**
Veterinary Voyeurs — PA	**163**
Helping the Ram Out — PJ	**169**
Trucking Lions — PA	**179**
Embarrassment at the Border — PJ	**185**
Far From the Madding Crowd — PA	**189**
Emil — PJ	**201**
Binky Boyle — PJ	**209**
The Telephone Call — PA	**215**
Beastly — PJ	**223**
Trusting Relationships — PA	**229**
Norwegians Would — PJ	**237**
Evolution — PA	**243**
Seen Yours Seniors — PJ	**251**
Wrapping Up — PA	**255**
The Final Curtain — PJ	**259**

FOREWORD

It is a real pleasure to write this foreword to Pete Anderson and Pete Jerram's new book *Old Dogs New Tricks*, and to acknowledge two veterinarians held in high regard by their clients and their peers.

If you are one of the many who read and enjoyed the original *Cock and Bull Stories* you will be looking forward with considerable anticipation to this new volume. If you haven't read the original, don't worry, read on, and then make sure you go back to the first volume. Like the first book, you will find this one disarmingly and refreshingly honest, with plenty of self-deprecating humour. Expect to be amused, entertained and enlightened.

However, this is not just a collection of amusing vet stories; it is also about what it takes to set up and develop a veterinary practice in a small rural town. The sheer hard work, the long hours, the pressures, the support from families, the fun, the enjoyment, and the resulting two successful veterinary careers.

These careers have seen both Petes become highly regarded by their peers, and at the forefront of their respective specialities of canine reproduction and sheep productivity.

So what exactly is it that vets do in their everyday work, apart from the obvious James Herriot-style activities of saving lives, dealing with sick animals, repairing broken limbs and mending damaged bodies? The reality involves tasks such as carrying out hundreds of rectal pregnancy examinations on cattle; tasks which inevitably come with entertaining stories, disasters and catastrophes.

As a country we seem to have been blessed with many agricultural fads, whether they be Angora rabbits, Angora goats, alpacas, ostriches, deer farming, fitch farming or fish farming. In this book you'll find out what was involved in providing veterinary services to these fledgling industries in these crazy times — and you'll enjoy the stories around them.

Veterinarians everywhere talk about the strong relationships they have built up with their clients over many years. Pete A and Pete J are no exception — in fact they epitomise why it is that rural vets have many fond (and not so fond) memories of a good number of their farmer clients. You will discover people of all descriptions: grumpy and cheerful, enlightened and not so, friendly and downright rude, hopeful and hopeless, as well as the pillars and the oddballs of society. You will also discover that the success of both Petes is down to their ability to truly understand their clients: their aspirations, their motivations, and their backgrounds. This over a cup of tea, or a 'wee dram', or even over a spell as opening batting partners in a social cricket game.

There is a limit, however, to what two individual vets can cover of their professional lifetime, and included in this book are a few experiences of other veterinary colleagues: from assisting a police manhunt to burning down a historic building to 'tooted elephants'.

This book will be read with interest for its insight into the changing face of veterinary practice in rural New Zealand over four decades. It describes how the profession has developed over these years to support agriculture as it has grown and diversified, and its accompanying successes and failures.

But at its heart *Old Dogs New Tricks* is the story of two friends and colleagues who have enjoyed their life as rural vets. The great deal of respect they have for each other, for their colleagues, for their families and for their clients shows through. Pete A and Pete J have both made significant contributions to their local communities and to the veterinary profession. And they've had a great deal of fun along the way.

Roger Marchant
Past President, New Zealand Veterinary Association
Waikanae
Kapiti Coast

WHY DO WE DO IT? — PJ

When Pete Anderson and I published our first book *Cock and Bull Stories*, in 2011, we really had no idea what to expect. Would it be ignored, laughed at, or seen as something worthwhile to country people?

One potential publisher had told us that our writing style was '1970s larrikin'. We nodded: Yes, she had that right. The book turned out to be a reasonable success, particularly with rural people, and those good souls were of course our intended audience. Most farming folk seemed to enjoy the stories, which was very gratifying. And we were lucky enough to be at number seven on the best-selling list for a couple of weeks, so we must have pleased some people. Probably 1970s larrikins.

There were some unexpected spinoffs. One farmer in the Buller catchment, usually fairly cagey about access to the river, recognised my name when I knocked on the door asking for permission to fish. Not only were we given access, we were offered use of his private farm road to get there — a generous act.

Another episode was not so gratifying. As a district councillor I was asked to give courtroom evidence as a non-expert witness in a major resource management case.

The legal counsel for the applicant, a gentleman whose name we won't bother repeating, decided he would attack my reputation. He produced a copy of Cock and Bull Stories and then proceeded to try to prove to the panel that the title of the book matched my character: that in fact I was, for want of a kinder term, a bullshitter. In a very public arena I was made to feel like the rabbit trapped in the burrow by the weasel. It was a gruelling and unpleasant experience that did nothing to build my admiration for those members of the legal profession who use the *ad hominem* method of cross-examination.

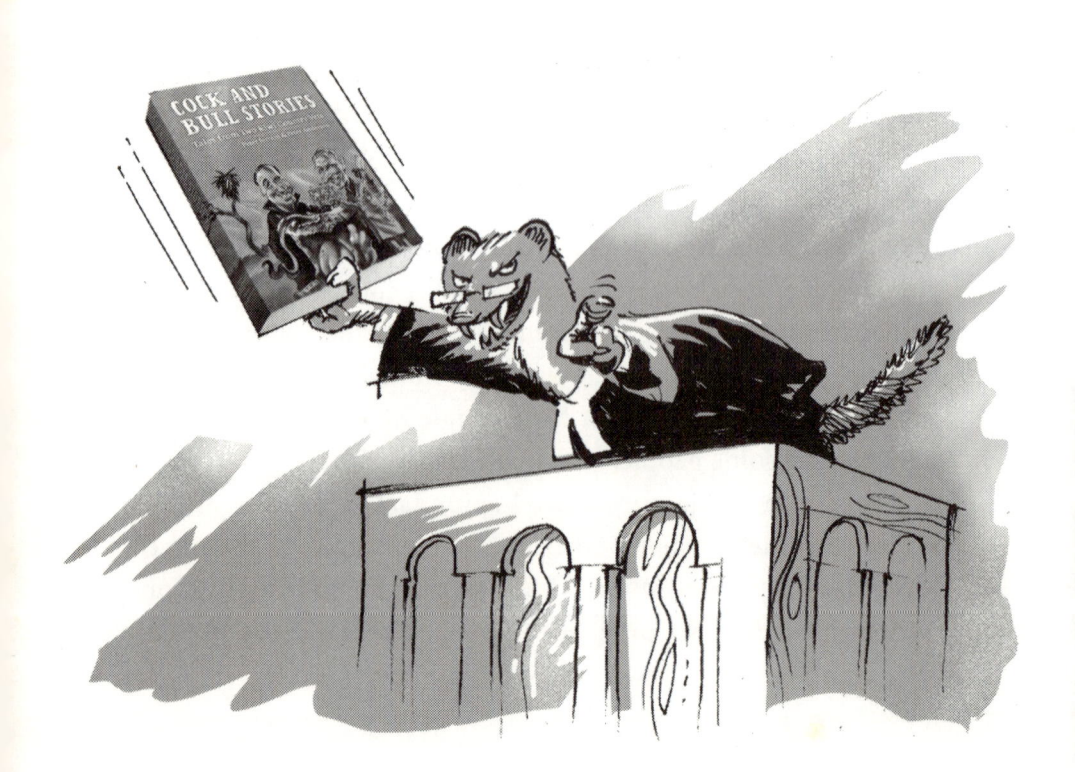

Even in 2016, five years after publication, I still get unexpected phone calls or emails from old acquaintances, employers, or total strangers, saying they've just discovered the book and have enjoyed it, and that's nice, and encouraging.

Soon after we wrote the first book we realised there were a lot more stories to tell. It's fair to say that I was more enthusiastic than my dear friend Pete A, but when Alex Hedley, from the newly amalgamated Penguin Random House, visited us, we agreed to meet a deadline and tell those stories.

Ally was always keen, and as before she is critic and supporter.

To Diane Thompson, my old friend and workmate for many years — thank you for your fast and accurate typing, and your ability to decipher my very bad writing. I'm sure that is a skill you have learned from your husband, 003.5 (retired).

And for our rural friends, we hope this book gives you some more insight into our lives as vets, the people we worked and (mostly) made friends with, and the wonderful region we live in.

I do hope I haven't offended anyone too badly in these stories. If I have, I apologise now.

I hope you enjoy *Old Dogs New Tricks*.

MY REASONS — PA

In 2011 Peter Jerram and I wrote and published *Cock and Bull Stories*, a series of anecdotes about our lives as veterinary partners in the wonderful province of Marlborough. After a few locals had read it some said to me, 'I've enjoyed your book, but why didn't you write about that time you came out and you were a bit late and everything went wrong and the bull wouldn't lie down and the horse kicked you? Gosh it was funny — but you weren't laughing.' So actually there was a good reason for forgetting some events but many of the stories people reminded me about I have again forgotten, mainly because I never for one minute thought I would be talked into writing a sequel.

However, Pete J is a persuasive character, and with Penguin Random House's encouragement I did finally agree that there was material for a follow-up book. I was also persuaded by a recent incident while on a flight to Auckland. I happened to be sitting at the rear of the plane, and on standing up at the end of the flight I noticed a woman in front of me with a copy of *Cock and Bull Stories* on her lap. I casually asked her if she was enjoying the book, to which she replied, 'Yes I am, but I'm really a little bit annoyed. I got the book to read on the beach in Rarotonga but I can't put it down and will finish it before we even get there.' She then looked at me and, I suspect in good part due to Ashley Smith's illustration skills, recognised a likeness. 'Why — are you . . .? Did you write this book?' she asked. I couldn't deny it, and so for a very brief moment I was a celebrity in the back of the plane. At least for her husband and two children.

So, yes, people did like *Cock and Bull Stories*. Many of the tales seemed to resonate with colleagues, and having known they would be our biggest critics it was reassuring that they too on the whole enjoyed the read. These colleagues, many of whom said they had a few stories to tell but admitted that they would never get around to writing a book, have contributed some yarns to this new volume. There are without doubt many more veterinary stories out there that also need to be written down. For most of us, our careers have been full of fascinating and exciting times, full of mishaps that we can now laugh about, full of achievements that we can be proud of, full of wonderful characters that have coloured our lives, and full of a huge range of animals with personalities of their own. All these are reasons why we vets continue doing what we do — and why, when we wake up in the morning, we look forward to the day ahead.

A TRUE GENTLEMAN – PJ

Weekends on duty, a major part of the lives of all rural vets, were not something I looked forward to. There was a lot of uncertainty, we never knew what was coming next, and in the first 20 years of our practice, there was no back-up on weekends.

No staff were rostered to answer the phone; our wives did that, valiantly, and at some cost to our families. And no staff were expected to be available to help in the clinic with emergency surgery. We did it all by ourselves, from administering anaesthetics to cleaning up the often considerable mess afterwards. And all the while the phone might be ringing, farmers or town people concerned about an animal. Weekends could be very stressful.

The jobs I enjoyed most in those days were the on-farm jobs, so when I received a call one Sunday morning from Alan Elliott, I wasn't too fazed.

'Hello, old boy. Are you the vet on duty?'

I was.

'Sorry to bother you, but our house cow is calving and it looks a bit tight. Can you come?'

Alan Elliott was a bit of a legend in the lower Awatere. A real gentleman of the English variety, he habitually wore a tweed suit and tie around the farm. His accent was very cultured and he lived by decent true Christian principles. Very much old school. I liked him.

Of course I could come, and minutes later I was off down the road in one of the two little Datsuns which Pete and I had bought when we started our own practice with no cash.

Brackenfield, the Elliotts' farm at that time, is just a few kilometres up the Awatere Valley, not far from State Highway One and about 20 kilometres south of Blenheim.

As I drove over the Weld Pass, separating Blenheim and the Wairau from the Awatere, the morning was fine and clear and the dew shone off the tussock-clad hills in the early spring sunlight. I felt good but, as always with a calving, a nervous anticipation was foremost. What would I find? A bit of lubrication and a firm pull? Perhaps one leg was back, or maybe there was a breech presentation which I could correct. Worst case would be a Caesarean section. We performed many of these on farm, but they took time, and a lot of concentration, and a strong capable farmer or farmer's wife could be a very helpful assistant.

As I reached the neat traditional house where the Elliotts lived, I could see the old gentleman waiting anxiously.

'Thank heavens you're here, she's getting a bit agitated,' he said.

I slipped on my overalls and went to have a look. She was a beautiful little Jersey cow, and I could see immediately that with a head and two front legs partially protruding from her rear end, this shouldn't be too difficult.

I pumped some water-based gel lubricant in past the calf and with a little bit of gentle twisting, and alternately pulling on one leg then the other, the calf started to move. There was a moment of hesitation as it reached mid-chest then a whoosh of fluid and I could lower the newborn calf to the ground.

Mr Elliott was delighted. 'That's wonderful, old boy. What shall we do with her now?'

I cleared the mucus from the calf's mouth, and made sure it was breathing. I gently pulled on the placenta and it came away easily. Good, sometimes they don't. For safety I slipped an antibiotic pessary into the now empty uterus. Assisting a calving can introduce a few foreign bacteria and this was standard practice. The cow could look after her calf now.

Mr Elliott was relieved and very pleased. 'Come up to the house, old boy, and clean up. We must have a sherry.'

It was 10 a.m. on a Sunday, I was half an hour from home, long before the days of cell phones. I had no idea what might be waiting for me at home. Guiltily, I said yes, I would come in, but only briefly.

After a wash up I was ushered into the sitting room. Lovely antique furniture upholstered in Sanderson linen adorned the room, among some nice mahogany pieces. I recall leadlight windows.

Mr Elliott sat me down, and from the sideboard produced a cut-crystal decanter. Carefully he half filled two crystal glasses with the dark sherry and handed one to me.

'Oloroso you know. Good stuff.'

I didn't doubt it.

'You've had a bit to do with our stud cattle, old boy.'

'Yes, I've calved a few cows, and I had to look at a bull for Alistair the other day,' I replied. Alistair was Alan's son, who lived on the property with his family and ran the farming operations now.

'Did you know that Brackenfield so and so came from such and such a family?' he asked, reeling off a long unfamiliar stud name, and I can't recall the particular name of the animal.

'No, I wasn't aware of that, Mr Elliott.'

'Oh yes, and of course he came from a line that you'd know well,' he said, running off another stud name.

I confess I know very little about the names of stud beef cattle but for half an hour I nodded wisely, murmuring the occasional, 'Yes, a wonderful line' or something similarly inane.

Mr Elliott was in seventh heaven. I think we'd gone back four or five generations by the time I'd finished my glass.

'Have another, old boy.' He was enjoying every minute of it.

'No, no, I really should go.' I was getting worried about Ally and the phone at home.

'Nonsense, I insist.' And he poured me a second glass as he launched into yet another generation of Angus bulls.

This time I gulped it down, as quickly as decency would allow at 11 a.m. on a Sunday.

'Thank you very much, Mr Elliott, but I really must be off.' I'd enjoyed my morning, but duty was calling.

'Well,' he said, 'that was marvellous. I don't often get to talk to someone who knows so much about Angus stud breeding.'

I had to cough to stifle my laugh. I had hardly got a word in and was really lost in his genealogy of the stud. I thanked him and Mrs Elliott, and drove off down the valley, feeling a warm glow.

Was it the sherry, or had I helped make an old man happy?

PREDICTABLY UNPREDICTABLE – PA

When I think back to all the amusing or embarrassing experiences I have had in my career the bulk of them seem to have occurred in my early days in the business. Other vets I have talked to also say the same thing. Is it because more of these memorable experiences actually happened then, or is it because these events took place during a very impressionable period in our careers?

Whatever the reason, those early days really were full of new experiences, and because of our inexperience there were far more opportunities for things to go wrong. We just had not been around long enough to appreciate all the consequences of what we were doing. And we had not yet fully realised that the only thing we could predict was the unpredictability of the animal and the outcome of the job ahead. Those early experiences, both good and bad, were often critical for driving the direction we eventually headed in our careers.

All this brings me to Mark Wiseman, who has a wonderful ability to laugh at his own misfortune and some amusing stories about his early days as a vet. Mark joined our practice in 2000. He had arrived back in New Zealand after practising in Britain for a few years and before that had graduated from Massey. Before coming to us he worked for a couple of years in Pahiatua.

While working on the Isle of Wight in the English Channel during his very early days in practice, Mark overnight became a famous arsonist. He had arrived at a farm to dehorn some calves with a gas-powered dehorning iron. However, to keep out of the hot midday sun the farm workers persuaded him that he should do this in the barn. Unfortunately there were no pens in the barn so the calves were running loose around him as he dehorned each one.

All was going well until one calf got its leg caught in the gas bottle pipe which yanked the burning iron from his hand. The iron then fell to the straw-covered floor which instantly ignited. To make matters worse the calf also sent the gas bottle flying, snapping the regulator off. The steady stream of gas escaping from the bottle turned it into a very impressive flame thrower, shooting out a flame about a metre long. Mark and the workers immediately evacuated the building. Fortunately all the calves had the sense to follow them.

This impromptu barn burning happened in a sleepy little village and it took a while for the local fire brigade to arrive. Mark waited anxiously for them, all the time expecting the gas bottle to explode, while the calves happily enjoyed their freedom in the field next to the barn. Fortunately for him the boss was away for the day and much to Mark's surprise the farm workers thought it was all a good laugh. When the fire brigade did finally arrive they were suitably impressed by the situation and sprang into action, building a make-shift pool into which they dropped the burning gas bottle. All the locals had gathered to watch and Mark became famous overnight as word spread very quickly on this small island. He thinks it was the most exciting thing that had happened in the village for a number of years.

The barn was a historic building but luckily had been made to last with solid stone walls and a slate roof. The only casualties were a couple of windows and some thick wooden rafters which were a bit charred. No doubt Mark, in future, would think twice about dehorning unpenned calves in a hay barn, even if it did mean working in the hot midday sun. He would also, after his next experience, learn that it's not just the unpredictability of the patient he had to be aware of but also that of the owner.

Mark got more than he bargained for when he was asked by his boss to make a house call to visit a sick cat. Mark thought nothing of the fact that the boss was trying to hide a smirk on his face. At his destination a middle-aged lady answered the door, holding her cat in her arms. Mark chuckles when he recalls her asking him if he had come to see her pussy. She ushered Mark in but as soon as he was through the door the cat decided to flee for freedom, scrambling up the lady's chest, over her shoulder and rapidly out of the cat flap. At this point the lady lifted her jumper right up exclaiming, 'Ooh! The little bugger just scratched my tit!' As she was wearing nothing under her jumper, not even a bra, Mark had to admit that yes, indeed, the cat had left a huge scratch all the way across her large breast! And as the cat was nowhere in sight Mark saw no need to hang around any longer and shot out the door himself.

Back at the clinic his boss asked how the house call had gone, this time unable to hide his smirk. It turned out that this particular client was well known for randomly exposing herself

Predictably Unpredictable | 25

and often requested house visits, a job usually handed over to the newest vet on the block.

While the rather traumatic barn incident quite possibly influenced Mark's future, encouraging him to avoid calves and horns and hay barns and farms, the experience with the escaping cat and its owner never stopped Mark from doing house calls or dealing with companion animals.

Bruce Taylor from Rangiora and I have followed similar paths in our careers. We both entered vet school together as the older students of our class, having had to complete other degrees before the powers that be let us study vet science at Massey University. We both started as general practitioners doing everything, but he eventually specialised in horse work, especially horse reproductive work, while I went almost solely into being a sheep and beef veterinarian.

Bruce knew it was time to drop the small animal work when he had to deal with a certain dog that really had him fooled. This New Year's Day encounter made him realise that his days looking after small animals were numbered.

He received a call at 3 a.m. from dog owners who reported they had run over their chihuahua-cross and that it was paralysed and unable to walk or stand. He got out of bed, dressed, went to the clinic and admitted the dog, where he confirmed that indeed it was unable to move. However, after examining the dog and finding all its cardinal signs normal and not being able to detect any signs of pain, he felt that it would be fine to leave the dog until the morning when he could give it a more thorough assessment and take X-rays if necessary.

This he did on returning to the clinic, and when he could find no obvious problems tried to see if the little dog could stand — not inside on the slippery floor but outside on the clinic lawn where it would have a reasonable chance of standing upright and moving.

This the little dog did in a very convincing manner when gently placed on the grass — he was off and away across the paddocks in seconds. Bruce gave chase but his hurdling of electric fences and leaping over ditches was not a patch on the dog's ability to run under and through them, and in minutes it had disappeared. Losing a paralysed dog is not easy to explain, and the day was spent putting announcements over the radio, endlessly calling around the vicinity of the clinic, and general hand-wringing. Bruce asked one of his partners, Gerry Stone, if his children (he and Jenny had a few) could go out and look for a very fast-moving white part-chihuahua dog. Around 7 p.m. he received a very welcome phone call — the dog had been seen but was proving difficult to catch. Eventually it was captured and discharged to the owners with the diagnosis of sore paws.

The owners eventually admitted that they had actually run over the dog on their way out on New Year's Eve at 7 p.m. but waited until they got home to call him. It was only then that they also told Bruce that the dog hated men. That, Bruce reckons, was the final straw — he had had enough of little dogs and some of their owners.

On the other hand good experiences tended to excite our interests and enthusiasm for areas of work. The 'insides' of animals always fascinated me. As a young boy I couldn't wait for my father to open up a hogget he had killed for mutton or an old ram for dog tucker and have a good play around with the innards. I guess it followed that I got very interested in doing autopsies on animals. Doing a post-mortem on a crook sheep can give an instant answer as to why the rest of the mob might not be thriving. I found this area of veterinary work fascinating and rewarding and became reasonably competent at it. Because of my interests, I identified for the first time in Marlborough — through thorough post-mortem examinations — certain diseases and deficiencies, and this was well before simple diagnostic blood tests were available. These included Johne's disease in sheep (a chronic debilitating fatal disease), bovine virus diarrhoea (BVD) in cattle, and iodine and vitamin E deficiency in goats and sheep. So it was natural for me to want to spend my time and efforts doing the stuff that turned my wheels: to work with mobs and herds and identify causes of poor health and performance and then help farmers implement management changes to improve production.

My fascination with looking inside animals was also a very good reason to get out of companion animal work. I would find any excuse I could to do an exploratory laparotomy on a cat or dog. In my companion animal days if I couldn't immediately determine what was wrong I wanted to open the animal up and have a look inside. This practice would nowadays be frowned on, and rightly so, but it did often give me instant answers. It amazed me, though, how many times I did an exploratory procedure and couldn't find anything untoward, but on recovering from the anaesthetic and fairly basic surgery an animal that had been mysteriously off-colour for months suddenly got much better. The only explanation I could give was that I had let the bad air out!

However, a desire to do exploratory laparotomies on companion animals or just do a post-mortem on them was definitely not good veterinary practice. It really was time I left these animals and their owners to the far more competent small animal specialists.

The opportunities available to new veterinary graduates are limitless and many vets end up doing the sort of work they never dreamed they would be doing during their university days. Chance and fate and early experiences all influenced which direction we took. Perhaps in the end most of us settled on the sort of work where we were most happy with the degree of predictability of the job. Some found the unpredictable nature of the work they were doing too stressful and had to change direction, while others revelled in the variety and intrigue and excitement. Large animal work tended to be far less predictable than small animal work, and that's what kept me interested.

AT THE BLUFF — PJ

The most common, and the most repetitive, job we ever did as sheep and beef vets was pregnancy testing cows. Most progressive farmers, and even a few who might not be described that way, see the necessity to check the cows, mostly in the first trimester of pregnancy, to see if they're in calf. There are several reasons for doing this.

First, an empty (or dry) cow is not going to produce anything to sell. She's also eating a lot of grass, energy that a pregnant cow could be putting into her calf. Another reason is that the autumn and early winter is a time when there's not a lot of cash coming in for most sheep and beef farmers, so the sale of any empty cows helps the bank balance. A final reason is that an abnormally high number of dry cows gives the farmer a heads-up that there's a problem. Is there an infertile bull, or a mineral deficiency? Is the farmer not feeding the cows enough or, worst of all, is there an infectious disease such as vibriosis (a bacterial disease of the reproductive tract) in the cows?

So pregnancy testing is a crucial part of the rural vet's life, and every autumn we'd begin to test, or PD (pregnancy diagnose), the herds in the district.

It's a tight breeding year for the average cow. Her pregnancy takes 275 days, she then has at least six weeks of post-partum anoestrus before she starts cycling again, which only gives her about 50 days at most to get pregnant if she's going to calve at the same time each year. She only cycles every 21 days, so she's got to get pregnant in the first or second cycle. Late calvers lead to all sorts of practical difficulties, and an uneven line of calves to sell, if that's the management on farm. It's important for all cattle farmers, beef or dairy, to have a fertile herd which more or less sticks to a schedule, and whose cows calve within a relatively narrow timeframe.

If all this is a bit tedious to read, I apologise, but it's a significant job and the practice of pregnancy testing led to a number of stories which we found pretty funny.

Marlborough is an extensive region, with long drives up and down dusty, blind-ended roads, and often long drives between properties, so we spent many hours on the road at PD time of year. I really enjoyed it. We were working with fine people who became our friends and the job itself was a good one, once you were fit for it. We did it all manually, and it was healthy hard work. These days ultrasound scanners have made the job much less physically demanding.

In my first year there was an element of anxiety. Like most new graduates, I hadn't done enough PD to be really confident, and I sweated my way through the first few herds. If I made any serious mistakes, I now apologise to those farmers, but no one ever accused me of doing so.

Later, it became very routine, but I still enjoyed it, yarning to the farmer, who was probably catching the cow's head in a crush and holding it while I shoved a lubricated gloved arm into the cow's rectum, and with my fingers palpated the uterus underneath it, through the rectal wall. A pregnant uterus contains fluid, and after about eight weeks of the pregnancy you can 'ballot' the foetus, that is, feel it bouncing in the fluid with the tip of your fingers.

One of my favourite places to go for PDs was Bluff Station in the Clarence Valley. The front country is in the Kekerengu Valley, 45 minutes south of Blenheim on State Highway One, but the bulk of the property lies out of sight of the casual observer, in the mighty Clarence Valley.

The Clarence River begins in the Molesworth/St James headwaters, not far from where a number of the big rivers of the northern South Island originate. The Waiau, Wairau, Clarence, and even the Buller headwaters all come from an area the size of one large station.

The Clarence then runs south towards Hanmer, turns eastward then northeast and courses between the two great Kaikoura Ranges, Seaward and Inland, before cutting out to the east coast at Clarence Bridge.

Bluff Station occupies a very large area of the more northern part of the river, and lies against the eastern side of the Inland Kaikouras, with the great mountains of Alarm and Tapuae-o-nuku the dominant land forms. We would test the cows at three or four different yards, at various places throughout this long station, usually 200 to 400 at each place.

One day, sometime in the 1980s, I left home early to go and test all the cows at the Bluff. I'd be away for two days, as it was a good three hours' driving from the homestead to the back yards at the Branch, the furthest outpost on the station.

I was, as always, excited to be going there. It's a magnificent wild place, and Chid Murray, the owner, is a good friend. Sue, his wife, has been a lifelong friend of Ally's too, so it was more than just a business trip. It was fun. Not many people get to see Bluff Station and I always found it a special place.

I was at the Glencoe homestead at Kekerengu by 8 a.m. and, I can't be sure, but I probably left my vehicle there and travelled with Chid in his 4WD Toyota. Or I might have taken mine. Over the hill we went to the major outpost of Coverham, where the married couple lived, about 45 minutes from the front. The road was windy and the going slow; in this modern world it took a special type of couple to live there. They did have power, and could just get TV, but otherwise they were fairly isolated.

At Coverham we picked up a couple of men, and in two or three trucks headed south, up the valley. Other men were already at the back of the station, mustering the cows. The rough road runs along the back of the Chalk Range, a long and steep limestone ridge which runs parallel as a sort of foothill range to the main Inland Kaikoura Range. A number of sizeable streams draining the range cut through the limestone, and each of these has to be forded, which isn't always possible in wet weather.

There is an outstanding geological feature of world significance here, one I knew nothing of in those days, and many times I blithely drove or was driven past it. At the Mead Stream a great twisted and curved limestone face, 200 metres high, has been exposed by centuries of river action. In the middle of this strata, a thick dark line, curved as the earth has twisted it, divides the face. The bottom edge of this dark line, where it transforms back to white limestone below is of great significance. It marks the K–T boundary, the exact year in which the Cretaceous period ended and the Tertiary began. This is one of many sites in the world where this phenomenon, identified by geologists in the late 1980s, can be seen.

At that point in time, 66 million years ago, a meteorite smashed into Mexico, causing massive and ongoing atmospheric dust, climate change and chemical change to the whole world. It was the event which led to the rapid demise of the dinosaurs and a chain of biological evolution which eventually saw the human race emerge as the dominant species on earth. The evidence is right here in Marlborough and of immense significance to our understanding of the history of our planet. But I knew nothing of this, as we crossed first the Swale, then the Mead and the Limburn, and finally the Dee, and climbed out to the Branch hut and yards.

It was a beautiful day and I can still see that magnificent landscape, the two great ranges, the men bringing a couple of hundred cows in from the holding paddock.

We had a quick bite of lunch, then I stripped, donned my overalls and apron/leggings, taped myself into two pairs of plastic gloves, and we were away. Chid was on the head bail catching the cows to hold them still, and I moved in and out of the vet gate, testing each one in turn, lubricating my arm every four or five cows to make the job easier.

Each time I pushed my arm in, I could turn my head just a little to the left and see the mighty peak of 'Tappy' high above. Chid and I yarned and the job was going well. Most of the cows were pregnant, but a number of young cows were often dry on the Bluff in those days. Chid was developing the country from rough scrub, and it was hard to find enough feed to give the first calvers the preferential nutrition they needed. The result was that a higher number of those cows didn't cycle in time to get pregnant second time around. It took a few years to beat the problem, but as the development kicked in, things got a lot better. At the time it worried Chid quite a lot, and I was very conscious of that. Pete A and I worked with him for several years to solve the problems, and his farm consultants were important to him too.

After about an hour, when I'd tested around 100 cows, the pen behind was empty. The men had gone off on horseback to get another mob up, so Chid and I went back to bring another yard full of cows up towards the race. I wasn't concentrating enough, and as we shooed 30 or 40 cows into the yard, I closed the steel gate a bit fast. The gate touched the hock of a cow and the laws of Newtonian physics were immediately realised as she kicked. Her hoof caught the gate at maximum velocity, the gate swung back violently, and hit me hard on the temple. I went down like a sprayed fly, and I can just recall lying in the mud, with cows running back over me, and Chid standing over me keeping me from further harm.

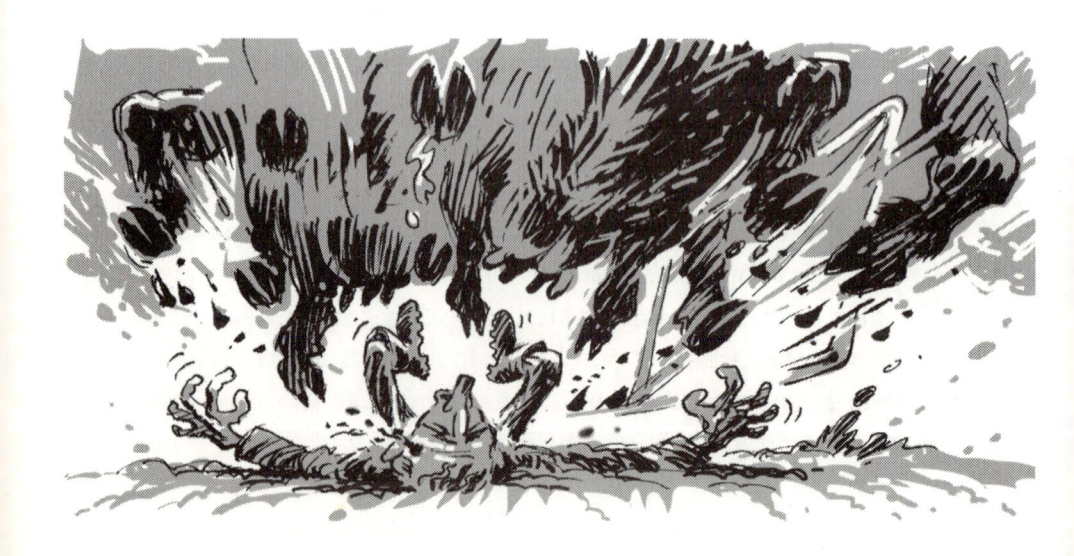

I think I must have been unconscious for a second or two, and I was a pretty sick boy as I clung to the rails of the yard, bleeding like a stuck pig from the wound over my right eye. I felt terrible, and Chid obviously didn't like the look of me. He was quickly on the two-way VHF radio in his truck. 'Bluff to Muzzle . . .' and in a few seconds Tina Nimmo at the Muzzle, a few miles upstream, was there.

'Pete's had a whack. He needs stitching. Can Colin take him out to Kaikoura?'

Colin could, and in half an hour the Cessna 180 was trundling up the airstrip half a kilometre away. I was bundled in beside Colin and we roared off across the valley, up, up and up against the Seaward Kaikouras, then over and down to Kaikoura's airstrip. At any other time it would have been exhilarating, but I wasn't in great shape and I didn't really appreciate it that day.

Colin and Tina Nimmo lived in one of the most inaccessible stations in the South Island, Muzzle Station. The only road access is either over the Inland Kaikouras then across the Clarence River in a difficult ford, or through Bluff Station on the track I'd come in on. When the rivers are up, there's no road access, but Colin has a helicopter as well as his fixed wing aircraft, and they're a hardy, self-reliant, cheerful and lovely couple. They have brought up their two daughters in fine fashion over the last 35 years, while farming a difficult place extremely well. It's now farmed by their daughter 'O' and her husband Guy Redfern, but this was well before their time.

At the Kaikoura airstrip one of Colin's mates picked me up and took me to the little hospital. The legendary Geoff Gordon, the town's long-standing doctor, was there. I was in my overalls, covered in cow manure, bleeding and dazed.

'That needs a few stitches, Pete,' he said, and in a few minutes had stitched me up.

'How long since you had a tetanus shot?' was the next question.

'I don't know, Geoff, a few years I think,' I mumbled.

'Well, you'd better have one,' he said, and without further ado stuck the needle of the syringe with the tetanus antitoxin through a layer of solid cowshit on my upper arm and pushed the plunger.

I was highly amused, if a little shocked. I thought maybe a bit of a wipe with meths on cotton wool might have been the thing. You know, for hygiene purposes.

Geoff was happily unconcerned. 'You'll be right. See you next time.' He grinned, and that was that.

We went back to the aerodrome, and half an hour later we were back at the Branch. Chid was concerned about the hold-up, but he could see I wasn't feeling great. My head, swathed in a wrap-around bandage, was splitting, and I wanted to be sick, and was.

So the job was postponed for the day, and instead of doing 300 cows at the Branch, and another 200 at the Mead yards, an hour down the track, we'd only done 100 for the day. The men did a few jobs, I went to bed, and at mealtime there was a bit of tension in the camp.

The next day was the hardest I ever did as a vet. I had a vile and constant headache and felt ghastly. But there was a job to do. With my heavily bandaged scone, I worked my way through the 200 cows at the Branch, then moved to the Mead, and did another 200. By then it was early afternoon. I had to tell Chid I needed food, so we stopped for a bit, but there were still another 300 at Coverham, another hour away.

I can just recall a pretty horrible three or four hours there, and by the time we were finished the sun was down. I drove home, sick as a dog, and spent the next day in bed. I'm sure I was concussed — I know Ally was a bit concerned.

But that experience didn't affect my great love of Bluff Station. I went there many times, both working and on hunting, social or climbing visits. On one trip five of us climbed Tappy, 2883 metres (9460 feet), from the Branch, camping on the tops the first night. Bob Rutherford was 75 at the time, and though he told Bill Lee, his son-in-law, to 'just cover me up with stones here' if he didn't make it, he got to the top and down safely.

It's a wonderful property, magnificent country, and I've always loved going there.

But I never forgot the Kaikoura tetanus shot — straight through the cowshit.

JUST DO IT — PA

As any young vet in a rural practice will know, dealing with emergencies and unpredicted jobs for which you have no previous experience is not uncommon. In the field you are suddenly faced with difficult situations for which no planning has been possible. You are on your own and you just have to make do.

I remember in my early days thinking of all the possibilities that might occur out of the blue, and I tried to be well prepared for any potential rare event. I had all the drugs and equipment I believed would be useful packed into my little Subaru, followed later by a second-hand and far too small Datsun Sunny. As a result I travelled the dusty back roads in a well-laden vehicle carrying too much never-to-be-used equipment and too many drugs that eventually had to be thrown out when they went past their use-by date.

As years passed, my cars got bigger and became air conditioned and more comfortable and I grew wiser and carried far lighter loads.

Anyway, with time, rural vets become fairly self-sufficient and invariably carry most things they are likely to require during a routine day. It's when we are suddenly removed from our 'office' and another means of transport is required to get to a job that we can find ourselves short of supplies and it becomes essential that we have the ability to improvise. In *Cock and Bull Stories* I wrote about one of the worst days in my life, at Molesworth Station, where halfway through castrating half a dozen unhandled three-year-old colts and after one had already died on me, another one herniated through the castration incision. I had to catch the colt in the middle of a large stockyard with his intestine dragging in the mud and re-anaesthetise with the remaining drugs and then clean and replace metres of filthy intestine before he came around. Having flown to Molesworth I didn't have any spare stocks of anything, so had to make do in a difficult situation. Having a horse herniate through its castration wound is an event you hear about during training but hope like hell you are never going to be faced with. They are not the emergency surgical events you can prepare for, but when they do occur you usually find a way to deal with them.

John Smart tells a wonderful story about being faced with an unusual situation in the Catlins when he was a very young vet, and barely a year in practice. It really illustrates how he adapted to the situation and helps explain why he has become one of the most well-known and widely respected sheep vets in the country.

The Catlins lie in the southeast corner of the South Island and contain the only area of native rainforest remaining on the east coast of New Zealand. Although well recognised nowadays, the Catlins were almost a forgotten corner of New Zealand when

John arrived in Balclutha in 1976. The main reason for this anonymity was the fact that the only way through most of the area was a very rough gravel road and getting into the depths of the country back then was regarded almost as a bit of an adventure. Because of their relative isolation, the farmers of the Catlins were a particularly hospitable bunch and always pleased to have a visitor to talk to. There is still a very strong community spirit in the Catlins.

In April 1977 John received a call just after lunch about a cut horse down at Ken and Shirley Mackenzie's farm at Chaslands, deep in the heart of the Catlins. The message was to meet at their house and they would take him to the horse, which was 'on a beach' somewhere. After an hour of thumping over endless potholes and corrugations John arrived at Ken and Shirley's. He was then informed that the horse was at the far end of Waipati Beach and getting to it would first involve driving in on the access road to the Cathedral Caves, a local tourist attraction. After arriving at the Cathedral Caves carpark he would need to collect all the equipment he might conceivably need and transfer it to packs on a horse. The horses would then be led down the winding pedestrian access track through native bush to the beach and once there mounted up and ridden 5 kilometres to the far end of Waipati Beach. Here they would have to cross the Waipati River and finally it was a short distance up onto a small plateau to where the patient was.

Horseriding was a novelty for John. As a classmate of his at Massey, I knew John would go to great lengths to avoid anything to do with horses. And he will admit to not having a lot of interest in matters equine. So he had only ever ridden a horse once before, as a small boy and reluctantly. This was to be his first real ride and it was 5 kilometres there and 5 kilometres back. Luckily the horse was a placid one and to John's relief behaved himself. It was a nice sunny afternoon and he almost enjoyed the 40 minute trek along the beach with the native bush on one side and the breakers of the South Pacific rolling in on the other. Due to lack of recent rains the Waipati River was not too high, and after fording it there was a short trek up onto a small grassy plateau above the river where John's patient stood by an old rusty one room corrugated iron musterer's hut.

Thankfully getting to our patients is not usually this involved. And while that part of the job was enough of an ordeal John then had to cope with his favourite animal, which had more of a problem than he had predicted. This horse had a very deep cut to the back of its front leg near the elbow. What had happened was Ken and Shirley had saddled up the horse with some equipment to go fencing. They had strapped a spade to the saddle and at some point the saddle had slipped causing the spade to dig into the back of its front leg.

It was an extensive wound that was going to take more than a sedative and local anaesthetic. Back then we didn't have the wonderful tranquilisers now available and so more often had to resort to a general anaesthetic to cope with difficult-to-stitch wounds. The most common drug we used then was an intravenous short-acting barbiturate anaesthetic — Thiopentone. The recovery phase from this could be long and wild. When you anaesthetise a horse you need a reasonable-sized area for the horse to fall onto but more importantly an area large enough for the horse to recover on. Getting to their feet in a groggy state means they stagger around a fair bit. Unfortunately for John, he only had the one small flat grassy area available, on two sides of which there were steep banks to the river below. John reckons he tried unsuccessfully to put out of his mind visions of a 'drunk' horse staggering off during the recovery phase and heading over the bluff and crashing onto the rocks in the riverbed below.

He organised the gear he would need and sedated and then anaesthetised the horse. It dropped to the ground with the cut leg uppermost, much to his relief. Ken, after one quick lesson, became an anaesthetist's assistant and, while John cleaned up the area round the cut and the wound itself, he sat on the horse's shoulder holding a syringe of anaesthetic in the jugular vein. Because Thiopentone only lasts for a short time the horse required several small top-ups to remain under for the duration of the surgery. And it would take some time to suture this mess back together again. When John sensed the horse getting a bit light he would get Ken to push a few more millilitres into the vein. John worked as quickly as possible because the more times you top up the longer and wilder the recovery phase is likely to be.

It was a challenging clean up and suturing job but once the surgery was finished and all the equipment removed from the vicinity then came the potentially tricky recovery. They waited quietly after the horse first started to stir, not wanting to disturb it — the longer it took for the horse to try to stand the better. Eventually the horse lurched to its feet and stood there wobbling. To John's relief it didn't try to take off. In the end the recovery he had been stressing over turned out to be somewhat of an anti-climax. The job ended up being a six and a half hour mission but a very successful one. The wound healed up well and the horse was back on normal duties within a couple of months.

After the long journey back John stayed for a well-deserved albeit rather late cup of tea with Ken and Shirley. During the course of the conversation the fact that John was marrying his girlfriend Lois in about a month's time came up. Before he knew what was happening Ken had loaded their old second-hand black and white television into his car. This was much appreciated since Lois and John didn't have two pennies to rub together but John says that this is typical of the friendly nature of the Catlins residents. This TV did exactly another two and a half years because John recalls it eventually died in November 1979 at the time of the Erebus disaster.

John had a demanding but memorable day, faced his fears, and was rewarded with lifelong friends and a TV set.

After dismounting at the end of that day back in 1977 John has never been back on a horse.

ANGORA ANGUISH — PJ

The 1980s were a time of significant change in New Zealand. The extraordinary social and monetary changes brought about by the Lange Labour government and its architect of reform Roger Douglas caused an unprecedented blossoming of apparent instant wealth among a middle New Zealand which had lived with austerity for generations.

Merchant banks (What on earth were they? we said) sprang up, cafés appeared on town and city streets, nightclubs and bars appeared or upgraded, and stayed open all night. People were able to borrow large sums of money, often with little security. You could borrow 70, 80, 90 per cent of the value of your house, something unheard of for our generation.

In the rural scene the nil standard value of livestock meant valuable stock could be bought and written down with huge implications for tax savings. It was meat and drink for entrepreneurial investors.

One by-product of that scenario was a huge surge in interest in Angora goats, which produce mohair, the lustrous fibre prized by some designers and manufacturers of garments. The mohair industry at that time was small, but almost overnight, purebred Angora goats, both does and bucks, became highly valuable, based on their scarcity and a lot of hype. At one stage bucks were selling for up to $100,000, and does up to $25,000: very large sums in 1986. Fortunes were made rapidly, and in many cases lost as rapidly later on.

With purebred Angoras being scarce, the question was: how to get more of those high-value animals? The veterinary profession found itself at the centre of the craze, for that is what it was. The answer, some believed, was embryo transfer. The drive came largely from city entrepreneurs, and a few country people who had Angoras already, and some others who saw it as a way of making a fast buck — no pun intended. In most cases, the hype and expectation turned out to be greater than the reality, but there were some successes, and they were very exciting times to be a vet.

Embryo transfer, or ET as it became known, involves treating the female animal during her reproductive cycle so that she produces not just one or two eggs, but many. If she is then inseminated at the right time by a top buck, the resulting embryos, potential little goats, become very valuable too. A doe can only carry two or perhaps three kids in gestation, but if the multiple fertilised embryos are harvested from her a week after mating, then transferred two at a time to surrogate does, they can be carried to full-term and produced as purebred kids. The result is that high-performing does may have 10 or 12 or more offspring in one year, rapidly increasing the quality of the Angora population and also providing high-quality animals for sale.

It's technical stuff, and while it might be old hat now, in the 1980s it was very much cutting-edge reproductive medicine, both in the understanding of the necessary treatments and in the very delicate surgery involved.

Our friend Roger Smith, farmer, rural banker and lateral thinker, rang us one day.

'What do you know about embryo transfer in goats?'

We didn't know much at all, but after a bit of prompting from Roger on how it would be good for us professionally to know how to do it, we agreed to find out. We could all make some money as well.

A few vets around the country had just begun to experiment with ET and Richard Lee, our vet friend in Waipukurau, was prepared to share his knowledge.

Pete and I flew to Waipukurau in a small aeroplane for the day, with experienced pilot Trevor Collins in the left seat, Pete A in the right, and yours truly perched queasily in the rear.

Learning new and interesting techniques was heady stuff and, with Richard's attention to detail, a good lesson for us. We travelled home in the little aeroplane, confident we could gear ourselves up and use ET to move a significant step forward, professionally and financially. We were broke, both with young families, big mortgages and a new business, so we definitely saw ET as an opportunity.

Roger had further plans. Errol and Jean Batty farmed Angoras close to Blenheim and were prominent players in the industry. They had won the coveted Diamond Fleece, the premium industry award, and were renowned for having good stock. Roger suggested we approach them with a view to using their goats, our expertise and Roger's land and premises for an ET programme.

Jean, a very good client, who had brought her business to

Anderson & Jerram when we set up, was a kind but pretty sharp-minded person. Errol, an accountant, was gentle and thoughtful but also a businessman. Convincing them to put their precious animals up for risky surgery wasn't going to be easy.

One evening we had a meeting at their house. Carefully, Roger outlined the plan. He would build a surgery to our specification, and provide the grazing and the practical management of the hormone programme. Pete A and I would provide the professional advice as well as the surgery, egg collection and transfer to recipient does. The Battys would provide the donor does, 12 of their best, and a high-quality buck. Roger, Pete and I would buy the recipient does.

The Battys would own 50 per cent of any resulting progeny, the Smiths and Anderson & Jerram the other 50 per cent. Then came the shock. The Battys wanted us to guarantee the life of the does, at a price of $25,000 each. A written guarantee would be necessary. This was a fair blow to us. At the time, our houses were worth about $35–$40,000 each, all highly mortgaged, and we had a large amount of bank debt in the business. Survival was a monthly challenge.

From memory, insurance was prohibitive, something like $2000 per doe for one month, at a value of $25,000 each. After a bit of nervous discussion we decided to take the risk, to carry the can individually. No insurance. The programme proceeded.

Roger built his shed and together we bought 200 feral does from a variety of sources. We designed the programme, bought the drugs and the necessary equipment, hired a locum vet for a month to run the practice and generally prepared ourselves, while Roger prepared the recipients to our instructions.

The Battys' does were programmed on their own place where Jean was more comfortable (as were the does) and they were to be brought out on the day. Pete and I had a couple of trial runs, doing the surgery and the flushing on feral does, so we would be comfortable and well practised on the day.

Roger had built a nice surgery, clean and hygienic, with a solid door between it and the viewing area. We couldn't have distractions at vital times during surgery, but Jean and Errol could observe through a small window.

The great day arrived. Pete and I were up early, vehicles packed, and we travelled out to the Smith farm with Jeanette, our surgery nurse. It was a crisp autumn morning in late April as we sped west to Renwick, then north across the Wairau River to the rough hill country on the North Bank. This country had been cleared by early settlers, first for gold and then for farming. The steep schist and semi-schist geology was not highly fertile, and was prone to erosion. From the 1960s the land was mostly abandoned farm grazing. Commercial forestry was planted on much of it, and gorse grew prolifically. Roger and Ket Smith had bought a small farm up a side valley west of the main road. The flats were productive, the hills planted in the ubiquitous *Pinus radiata*. It was colder in the valley than the Wairau Plain, which we'd just left, as we wound up the gravel road to the surgery, a converted woolshed. We were a bit tense as we set up our anaesthetic gear and laid out our sterile surgical equipment and the flushing equipment. There was a lot at stake for us.

The Battys arrived with the first six does. We would do the next six tomorrow. Jean was very tense, while Errol attempted to settle her anxieties with gentle words. It was Pete A's job to anaesthetise the does for surgery, and intubate their larynxes with tubes made for the job. This meant we could maintain the anaesthetised state with gas, far safer than topping up with the drugs used to induce. In humans, dogs, and even cats, this intubation is pretty straightforward. The anaesthetist can easily visualise the larynx and the arytenoid cartilages at the back of the throat, marking the opening to the trachea. But for sheep and goats (and deer) it is much more difficult. The larynx is a long way back, and the natural curve downwards makes it very hard to visualise. A special long curved laryngoscope, complete with battery-powered light, is absolutely necessary to intubate and even then it's a tricky business.

Pete injects the Pentothal into the jugular vein of the first doe, who falls instantly unconscious. While Roger holds the doe's head, Pete carefully intubates her and blows up the cuff. This means that should she regurgitate rumen contents, they can't run into the lungs.

Pete and Roger quickly clip her belly to the skin and bring her into the surgery, where I await, fully gowned and gloved in sterile gear. They place the doe belly up, head down on the steeply sloping surgery table. The slope means her intestines will slide forward making the uterus easily accessible for surgery.

After Jeanette has sterilised the skin with iodine and alcohol, she passes me a sterile drape, which I place with its rectangular hole over the surgery site. The intubated goat is connected to the anaesthetic machine, which will supply oxygen plus anaesthetic gas during surgery.

We proceed. Carefully I cut the midline skin just forward of the udder, an incision of about 6 or 7 centimetres. Then, even more carefully, I make a small incision in the connective tissue and the lining of the gut, the peritoneum. Using scissors, I expand the cut. We are in! Gently pushing aside the fatty omentum, I expose the shining, glistening, pink uterus, looking like two curled-up fingers which unite as the body of the uterus further back. With some gentle movement of tissue, I find the left ovary at the forward end of the left uterine horn and oviduct. Manipulating it with a blunt probe, I carefully turn the ovary over. It is about the size of the end of a thumb, but what I'm interested in is counting the corpora lutea on it. Each corpus luteum is a small bulging raspberry red protrusion on the surface of the ovary, signalling where an egg was shed seven days ago when the doe ovulated. By counting the corpora lutea on both ovaries, I get a good guide to how many eggs we should find when we flush her.

I don't recall the numbers. There may have been four on one ovary, six on the other in that first doe, a total of 10. So we expect 10 fertilised embryos.

Then Pete A hands me the Foley catheter. This is a 15-centimetre-long catheter with two holes in the top, for collection, a wide mouth at the other end for passing the harvested fluid and a cuff to be blown up with air or fluid, just behind the collected holes. This ensures all the fluid goes through the catheter, and all the embryos are harvested.

I push a hole in the left uterine horn near the bifurcation with a pair of artery forceps. Then I introduce the catheter, nose first, and pass it into full depth. I carefully blow up the cuff using a syringe full of saline. This is a critical procedure. Too tight could rupture the uterus wall, rendering the doe permanently infertile; too loose means we lose the embryos. Gently I blow it up until I'm satisfied it's firm. That will work.

Pete then passes me the flushing fluid in a 20 millilitre syringe, and a plastic tom cat catheter. I find the ovary, then probing gently, I pass the catheter past the fimbriae: the 'fingers' which are the beginning of the oviduct and which would normally collect each embryo as it leaves the ovary to enter the oviduct on its way to the uterus. With the catheter successfully in the oviduct, I attach the syringe of flushing fluid, while Pete A waits with a petri dish at the open end of the Foley catheter. I begin to inject the fluid.

Pete reports on progress: 'Drip, drip, drip, drip.'

We need a good flow to get the eggs flushed out of the uterus, not a drip. Eventually I hear 'Good flow' and I press harder on the syringe until all the fluid has passed through the uterus, through the catheter and into the petri dish.

Pete then places that dish of embryos very carefully on the microscope as he readies to count for eggs. I wait. After 90 seconds he finds one, then others.

'Six,' he says.

Satisfied, we then follow the same procedure on the other side of the uterus. Four there. A good harvest.

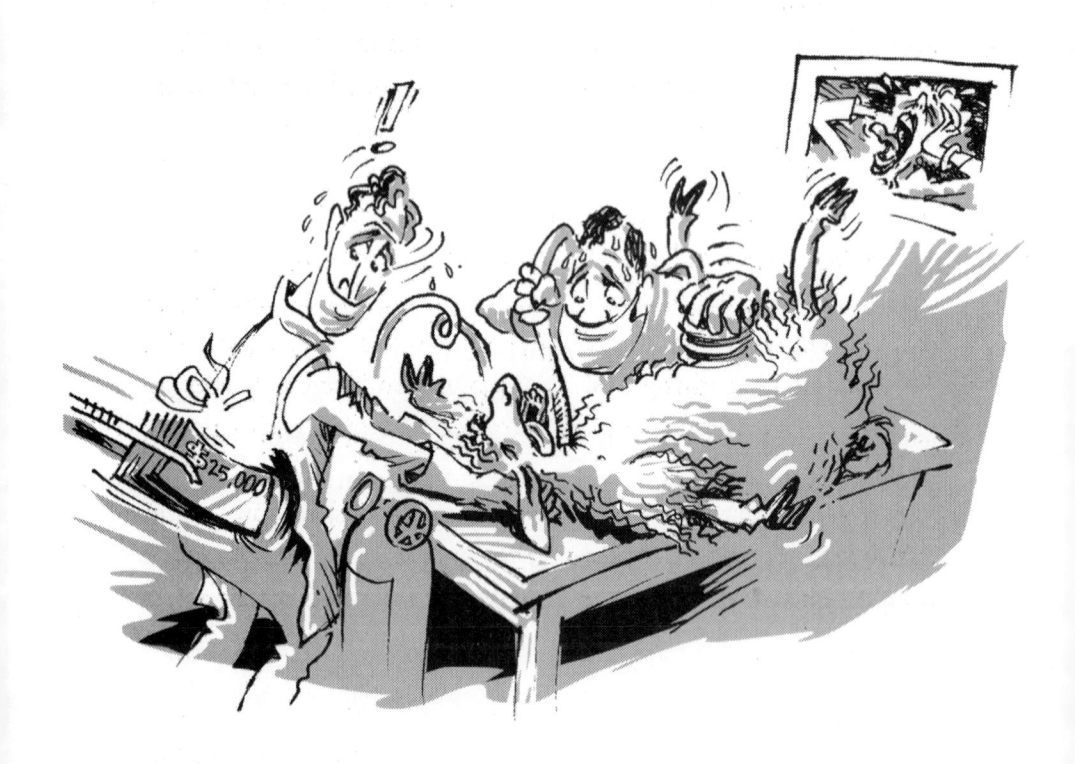

It is tricky, demanding work that requires a lot of concentration, and we are aware of Jean peering anxiously through the viewing window. Eventually we are done. I suture the doe up, then Pete and Roger take her out to recovery, where Jean and Errol can look after her.

The doe receives a shot of antibiotics, and when she starts to swallow, the tube is removed. We carry on, and do the same on the next five does. The results are variable, between 12 and zero for each doe. I think we average six or eight embryos per doe. A reasonable result.

In the afternoon we transplant the harvested embryos, two at a time, into the recipient does.

In that first season we did all that part surgically too, which made for some long and exhausting days. In subsequent years I developed skills using a laparoscope, so we only had to sedate the recipients and use local anaesthetic at the entry sites. This was much faster and easier on the animals. But this first year we were still learning.

The upshot was a fairly successful first day. Jean was relieved, and she and Errol took their precious does home for some TLC.

We went home and slept well. So far, so good. The following day we repeated the whole procedure. The first donor doe came with a warning. 'We got this one from Rae Adams. It's always held its head to one side a bit,' said Jean.

Pete injects the Pentothal and the doe goes to sleep. Then disaster. The problem comes when he tries to intubate it. He just can't find the larynx. Sweating a bit, but still calm, he keeps trying. The goat isn't breathing, and its mucous membrane begins to go very blue. All I can think of is the $25,000 we will have to fork out, a sum that will ruin us.

With me on the verge of panic, and Jean shouting, we get the dying doe onto the table, and with minimal preparation I pierce a hole in the larynx from the outside, a tracheotomy. Pete shoves the tube into the trachea, we blow up the cuff and begin ventilating with oxygen, squeezing on the bag to inflate the lungs. We can hear Jean shouting from the viewing area. It was one of the worst moments of my veterinary life.

After a few minutes pink colour was returned to the doe, and eventually she breathed on her own. But we weren't going to risk her and removed her from the programme. It was a close call.

After a breather we carried on. The next doe was uneventful and produced six embryos. The third one was also going well. I was just starting to flush the uterus for the first collection when there was a banging on the window.

It is Jean who then bursts through the door.

'That doe isn't breathing!' she shouts.

Our nurse Jeanette is monitoring the breathing, and has an audible beeping alarm to help. This will go off after 30 seconds. It is now about 24 seconds. As Jean comes in, the goat breathes. This time we are grumpy.

'You are compromising the success of this operation, Jean,' I say. 'Please leave!'

She did and we carried on, but it was another dicey moment.

I am pleased to say that we remained good friends with the Battys and when Jean died some years later, the family even invited me to speak at her funeral, a task I accepted humbly and with pleasure. At the funeral I recounted the incidents with the goats, and Jean's anxieties, which surprised no one.

Jean was a wonderful person, strong, dedicated and loyal, and she had a huge passion for her animals and the mohair industry. We were very fond of her. But she could be a challenge to those of us who provided professional services.

FOOTNOTE

After three or four years, the ET craze died out quickly with goats, but the training allowed us to do a lot more in both deer and sheep ET in the years to come. It was a defining and developmental phase of our professional careers, and we raised our standards considerably, both technical and organisational — things which stood us in good stead from then on.

HOOF TO PROPELLER – PA

Rural vets are totally dependent on their vehicles to do their work. Rarely do our patients come to us so our cars or utes become our offices. While many vets have preferences for a particular shape or make of vehicle they all have one thing in common. Inside, they all smell the same. It's a combination of drugs, antiseptics, used overalls, wet boots, the odd bit of animal tissue gone bad and ruminant faeces. We get used to the smell but our families never seem to.

We have to cover a fair bit of ground on our house calls, so we spend a lot of time sitting behind the wheel. My car is my communication centre. By cell phone or radio-telephone I keep in touch with the rest of the practice and the radio keeps me in touch with the rest of the world. It's also my entertainment centre. Long trips are helped by having good music in the background. As I've said the car is my office. Materials used at the last job and mileages to the job are recorded before I head off to the next farm call. A tape recorder to note thoughts or advice for the farmer that might come to mind while driving are also part of some vets' office equipment. Too often the front seat is also my cafeteria. One of the joys of large animal practice is actually being able to relax after a morning or afternoon's work, having a cup of tea and bite to eat with the farmer and family. But often I am running late and it is 40 minutes' drive to the next call, so I forgo that pleasure and eat a sandwich or apple and drink my thermo-cup of lukewarm tea on the way.

When I was in full-time clinical practice anyone looking through the driver's window undoubtedly thought 'what a mess' — notepad, day diary, record forms, prescription pad, certification pads for different contingencies scattered all over the floor and passenger seat and intermingled with an apple or two, water bottle, used thermo-cup, reading glasses, cell phone and a couple of parcels to drop off at farms on the way. In the early days my bull terrier mate Roo enjoyed snuggling among this collection of everyday requirements, things that needed to be within arm's reach. And anyone looking into my boot would have thought 'what a shambles'. The boot was my workbench and storeroom and I knew where everything was. It might have taken a bit of shifting of boots and bottles to get to an infrequently used piece of equipment but I always knew where to go.

So in a funny sort of way I got quite fond of my vehicle, and when I had to abandon it and use another means of transport to get to a job, as was not infrequently the case, I felt as if I didn't have a mate along for the ride. However, with all the different cars I have had over my 40 years of veterinary practice none have meant as much to me as the aeroplanes I have flown and used for work. Perhaps it is the sheer thrill I get out of flying but in fact it is more than that. These planes have all given me moments of excitement, fear and pain, as well as spectacular and unique scenery and wonderful peace.

I first started flying soon after graduating and coming to work in Marlborough. At that time the Graham Veterinary Club frequently used the local Marlborough Aero Club to fly vets to various far-away jobs. Often it meant the pilot had to hang around all day while we did the work although they were in many instances very useful vet assistants. As I had always wanted to fly it seemed the logical step for me to get my pilot's licence and then see if I could actually fly myself to the jobs. Once I did get my private licence, I could understand and appreciate why the Marlborough Aero Club was reluctant to let an inexperienced pilot take its planes into remote back-country airstrips. I really needed to get some experience with my own plane, where there were no restrictions on where I went, and in 1985 I became a quarter owner of a 90HP Piper Cub BQX. While it was a delight to fly it was very light and had the horrible tendency of wanting to fly even when I wasn't in it. In the very slightest of breezes BQX needed thorough tethering to the ground whenever I left it to do any veterinary work. BQX was sold after a year and I next became a half-share owner in a Piper Colt EEW. While this two-seater was underpowered and had limited short take-off and landing (STOL) characteristics I gave myself more scares and thrills in it than any other. It was the machine in which I really learned to fly in the mountains. Unfortunately it all came to an end when I crashed on landing on a farm strip in Kekerengu (see 'Flying and Work' in *Cock and Bull Stories*).

After EEW was wrecked and I had recovered from a rather nasty knock to the head I flew one of the world's favourite back-country planes, the Piper Super Cub. BPG was owned by Lands and Survey who owned Molesworth Station, but it was kept at

Omaka near Blenheim and managed by the Marlborough Aero Club. It really was a delight to fly and a very practical machine to use for veterinary work in the back country. However, it too had a sad ending when it blew over and was wrecked one night. Although I had tied the plane down well behind the super-bin on a topdressing strip on Mike and Kristen Gerard's property in Clova Bay in the Marlborough Sounds, it blew over in some severe squally wind conditions. I had overnighted on Pohuenui Station in the outer Sounds, having gone there by boat. As we came into the jetty on returning to Clova Bay, I could see wheels rather than wings outlined against the super-bin. Not a pretty sight and as she was the favourite plane of all pilots I was definitely not Popular Pete at the aero club after that.

For the last 20 years I have been flying an ex-topdressing plane, a Piper Pawnee CIQ I bought off a local ag pilot Ray Patchett. While it is slow and uses far too much fuel it has heaps of power, a large hopper which can carry lots of equipment as well as three jerry cans of spare fuel, and copes well with short rough farm airstrips or paddocks. Another advantage of having a hopper is that I do not get clouted in the back of the head by airborne pieces of equipment when I get into turbulence — a not infrequent event in my other planes. I find it ideal for the job and love flying it.

Because of Marlborough's topography, with several mountain ranges separating fertile farmed valleys, an aeroplane has been indispensable. Often I will do a full day's work from the plane, involving several calls and far more than would be possible by driving. However, unlike the car where I have learned to carry most things for most contingencies, when flying I do have to think of everything I might need for the day and what to take out of the car and put into the hopper before taking off. On a few occasions I have forgotten important pieces of equipment, including basics such as gloves and lubricant when pregnancy testing cows, and emasculators when castrating horses. You just make do. On another occasion I didn't take enough Tuberculin to TB test a deer herd. I really couldn't make do then and had to fly back to town for more, an hour and a half round trip.

So for rural practitioners our vehicles, whatever they may be, are a vital piece of equipment and absolutely essential for the job. Surprisingly, unlike some urban professionals with super-smart 4WD SUVs, which seldom get out of 2WD, no rural vet I know gets too sentimental about his vehicle.

DON'T BITE THE HAND — PJ

We vets have a sometimes risky job. All professions have their associated hazards, but I can't think of many which require a university degree and also have such a high physical risk. Dealing with large animals always carries some danger and PA and I talked about some of our moments with deer, cattle and even merino rams in our first book. We understand the perils, and the boundaries that we shouldn't cross, but sometimes have to.

But companion animal vets can come up against it too, as I found out a few times in my career. I'm not going to talk about cats; an angry cat is a very dangerous animal, but all vets face this.

An angry or scared dog though is another story and I want to share some of the best, or worst, of those tales.

Old Mr Yealands was an interesting and thoughtful chap, and when he brought his corgi, Rex, into the Graham Veterinary Club in my second year after graduation, I welcomed him, and ushered them both into the consultation room.

Companion animal medicine was very much secondary to farm animal medicine at the vet club, and the facilities were adequate, but not like today's modern clinics. I'm sure the smell of that old clinic engendered a lot of unease and fear in a lot of dogs, and Rex was no exception. It was also the time when parvovirus first reared its head in New Zealand. We'd been reading about the nasty enteric effects of this disease for a year or two in American and British veterinary publications, and the first cases had begun to appear in New Zealand. It's a terrible condition, attacking mostly the intestinal tract, and when the virus first arrived here there were many sad and devastating cases, mostly in young dogs. Those who were around then will never forget the characteristic smell in the kennels of those retching, scouring animals, and the horror of their owners as their precious pets suffered and died.

Within months of the appearance of the disease a vaccine arrived, and a new era in companion animal veterinary medicine had begun.

People who had had no contact with vets literally queued at clinics to have their dogs vaccinated, and the subsequent awareness of what a vet could do led to a sudden and permanent rise in the fortunes of small animal vets. But this was in the future.

'What can I do for you, Mr Yealands?' I asked politely.

'Old Rex needs a vaccination, and you'd better have a look in his ears too. He's shaking his head a bit.'

Aha, I had two things to do. This would be a good consultation.

'Hello Rex,' I said, and bent down to give him a pat. Without warning the old corgi leaped at my extended right hand and bit savagely, his upper and lower canine teeth almost meeting in the soft flesh between my thumb and forefinger. I looked at the deep and ugly wound, at the blood pouring from it and I am ashamed to say adrenaline, anger and shock took over.

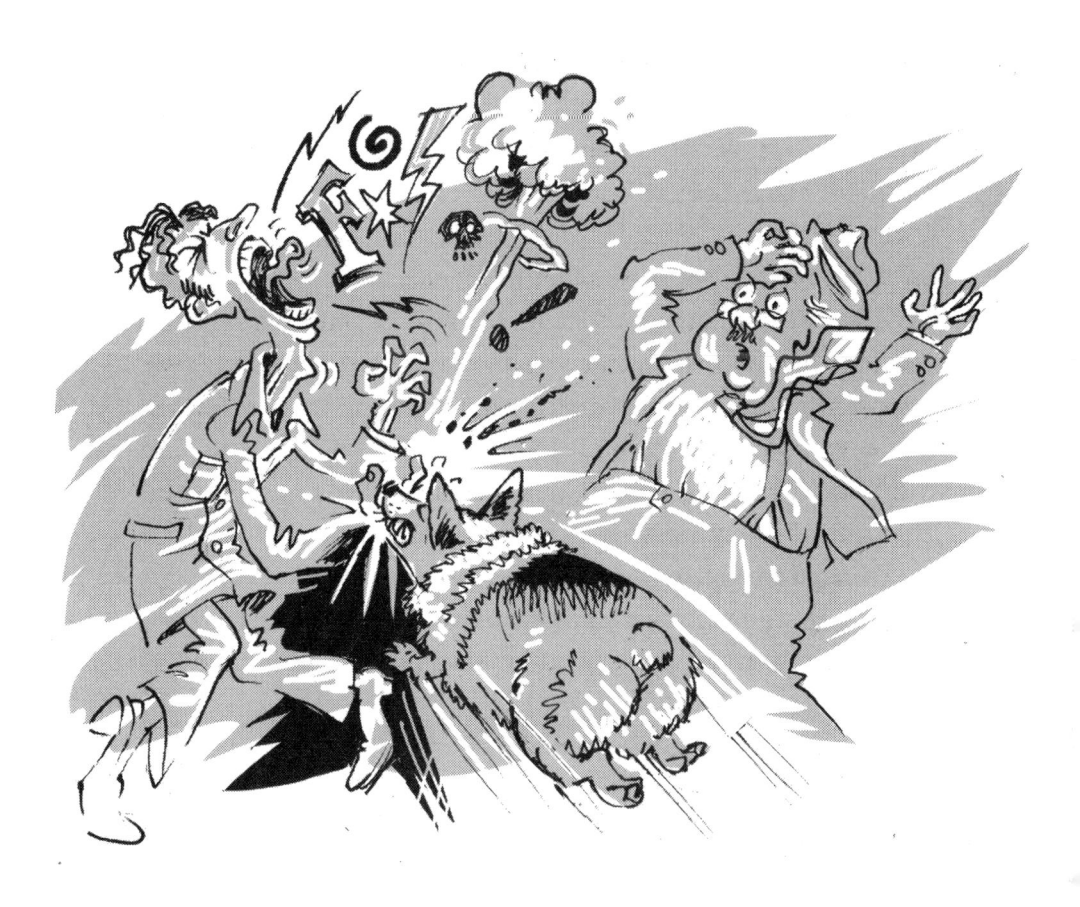

'Fuck!' I shouted, rattled to the core.

Now if you think that doesn't sound very professional, you're absolutely right. But just occasionally, in the heat of the moment, we can all let ourselves down a bit, as I did then. I was embarrassed at my oath, but shocked and in some pain.

'He doesn't like strangers,' said Mr Yealands.

Thanks.

It took the nurses 10 minutes to clean and bandage my hand,

and I think one of the other vets asked the owner to muzzle old Rex, then did the required examination and vaccination. My hand, the precious right one, was out of action for a week, then the incident was forgotten.

But there was a humorous sequel. Three years later, after PA and I had left the vet club and set up in our own private practice, Anderson & Jerram down the road, I saw in the consultation book that a Mr Yealands was booked in during the morning. It was the same gentleman. He had a different dog, a nice-natured corgi that was quite happy to greet me as most dogs do, allowing me to pick it up and put it on the examination table. I finished examining the little animal without ever mentioning the incident with Rex.

'Nice to see you here, Mr Yealands,' I offered.

'I used to go to the vet club,' he replied, 'but there's a vet there who used the most foul language the only time I went, and I'm never going back!'

I was ever grateful the dear old chap had failed to recognise me.

Another even more dangerous dog which I saw years later at The Vet Centre became almost a friend, although not without our exercising great care in our handling of him.

Kramar was a German shepherd, but not just any German shepherd. He was an official New Zealand Police dog in the care of Constable Richard van Asch.

Richard was an old friend of ours. His family were clients, and as a schoolboy he wanted to be a vet. I encouraged him, but he found the academic subjects hard going, in particular physics. He spent a bit of time with PA and me in those years and we watched with interest when he won an AFS Scholarship for a year in Greenland, of all unlikely places.

He got a pretty tough placement too, his first family having no spare rooms or beds, so Richard slept on a sledge in the living room after everyone else had gone to bed. It was a hardening experience for Richard and when he came back he joined the police, and became an excellent officer, and a dog handler.

I can't recall how many dogs he'd had before Kramar, but he was very proud of this very hard dog. Quite a few felons had felt the grip of Kramar's fangs. This dog had a real attitude. All humans were fair game, if Richard said so.

When we handled Kramar in the clinic Richard always put a muzzle on him first, but even then he had to hold the dog very firmly if we were doing anything to him such as vaccinations. Blood-curdling growls would emanate, and he meant business. When he came to stay for a day, needing some procedure to be performed, he would be put in a large cage, like other dogs. But whenever anyone came into the kennel room Kramar would rush at the cage door roaring and gnashing.

The solution was a bunch of keys on a large ring, which Constable Richard always left with us. You only had to pick them up and give them a shake, and Kramar would instantly sit quietly, allowing the vet or the nurse to clip a lead on him and take him into the surgery. It paid to carry the keys with you.

Kramar was such a good police dog that the powers that be wished to use his genetics. They wanted him to be a sire. But he had a wee problem. Kramar had a condition known as priapism.

When he had an on-heat bitch in front of him for services, his erect member would be painfully strangled by the too-tight opening of his prepuce. It made mating a very painful process for Kramar, and worse, he was convinced it was the bitch he was serving who was causing him this terrible pain, so he'd chew into her. He inflicted real damage on some good German shepherd bitches.

The police handlers in Wellington wanted a solution to his

problem, but they also wanted Kramar's semen collected and frozen in case any surgical remedies for his physical shortcoming weren't successful. I told Richard that if he wanted Kramar to be a successful stud, or even wanted to collect semen from him, the dog needed surgery to increase the size of his preputial opening.

On the day of surgery, Richard stayed with the dog while we anaesthetised him and laid him on the table. It was a delicate operation. If I took too much off, the opening would be so large that his willie would hang out of it all the time. That could lead to damage and infection. If I didn't take enough, we wouldn't have achieved anything.

I had to judge the correct amount for an erect member to comfortably protrude, and of course it wasn't in that state when I did the surgery.

I'm happy to say that the surgery was reasonably successful, and later on I did collect and freeze some of Kramar's semen. I think I used all dissolving sutures too, so we wouldn't have the slightly dangerous job of removing them. It was always a mildly nerve-wracking business handling Kramar, but he became quite a friend in the end. And I would never have wished to be the felon he latched on to.

There were also a few dogs who we just couldn't trust, and it nearly always came down to their owners. There are some people who shouldn't own dogs. They are the ones who are unable to grasp that you have to be firm, be the leader of the pack. This can be easily imprinted on pups from a young age with good training, and for those dogs, and their owner, life is usually stress free. But many can't understand the principle. Those people's kids are usually undisciplined as well.

One nice young woman brought her one-year-old Rottweiler

in for castration. The dog seemed fine after she left him, but that particular breed is not one I've ever trusted, so when we brought him into surgery we handled him with care: friendly and calm, but firmly.

As the nurses held him, I made to lift his paw to inject the intravenous anaesthetic. Without warning the dog lunged at my face with a savage snarl, teeth cracking together as he tried to get me. We took another tack, gave him a heavy sedative by subcutaneous injection, then managed to get him anaesthetised and castrated.

When the owner came to get him she brought her partner.

'Can I have a talk?' I asked, and they followed me into a consulting room. When I told the young woman that she had a potentially dangerous dog she flew off the handle.

'He's harmless. You don't know how to handle him!' she shouted.

I explained that I'd been doing this for 30 years, that I enjoyed working with dogs, but this one was going to give her trouble. She would have none of it, but her partner was more detached.

'He's right, you know, Liz,' he said. 'He's pretty funny around a lot of people.'

The woman eventually listened and even gave me a slightly friendly smile as she left. I heard later that the dog had badly bitten someone and had been euthanased. It was a case of wrong dog for that owner.

Vets have a saying: 'There are no bad dogs, just bad owners.' It's a pretty fair call although there are a few breeds of dog which tend to be less trustworthy than others — Rottweilers and chihuahuas are examples. But dogs are pack animals, and they will respond to a strong leader. That's where good behaviour comes from.

As I write, there's a fantastic TV show featuring animal behaviourist Mark Vette. He's a real pro, and I love watching him deal with all the problems I've seen in my career. But the overriding message is to start them young and teach them that you, the owner, are the leader of the pack. If you train them before they're four months old, you've got a well-behaved dog for life.

Mostly . . .

A LONG DAY ON D'URVILLE — PA

Pete J always told me I was a very poor risk assessment judge. By the end of this one day on D'Urville Island I had proved him right.

I always looked forward to my visits to D'Urville Island, not only because of the friendships I'd developed with the three farming families there but also because of the unique and beautiful landscape. Early Maori also valued this island. It is exposed to the winds but is warm, has a plentiful supply of kai moana at hand and is one of the few sites in the country where rare and valuable argillite can be found. Maori valued argillite's strength, hardness and ability to hold a sharpened edge, ideal for making adzes. Both Patuki Station and Waitai Station have pa sites overlooking the coast with an uninterrupted view of Cook Strait and the North Island. Further south can be found the old Maori argillite mines. The whole island has a number of very interesting sites to explore.

However, getting to the island, which lies at the northernmost tip of the Marlborough Sounds if coming from the mainland, requires at least three different modes of transport. Driving to French Pass from Blenheim is a good two hours, next a water taxi or barge gets you to the island with all your gear, and then you jump into an old van that's been left at the pier, again with all your gear, and drive yourself to one of the three larger properties on the island. Often all three. It's another hour's drive to the tip of the island where Gus and Bex Forgan manage Patuki Station. So it's eight to nine hours of travel each round trip, and as a result I would often stay overnight with one of the families. Over the years I have spent many an enjoyable and entertaining evening with Gus and Bex and their three amazing young daughters, or with Shayne and Pam Amyes and their daughter on the next-door property Waitai Station.

The farms on D'Urville Island are probably more akin to North Island farms than the typical Marlborough farm. The hills are steep but clean and well grassed. On D'Urville there is always the constant sound of the sea in the background and the views are amazing — Stephens Island of tuatara fame to the north, Nelson Bays to the west, and the North Island to the east. However, it is exposed to winds and that natural feature plays a significant part in my story.

As you can imagine when going to D'Urville Island I prefer to fly. Forty minutes from home and forty minutes back. But one day this journey took a lot longer and in the end required several modes of transport.

It was early summer and a ram testing day was planned along with a number of other little jobs on all the properties, including dog vaccinations, a lame horse and animal health programme updates. First was Waitai Station, then Patuki and then I was to fly down to Greville Harbour near the southern tip of the island where Steve and Janet Norton managed Ragged Point. Getting to the Nortons' involved a 10 minute walk from the airstrip to the beach in Greville Harbour and then a 10 minute boat trip across the bay to Ragged Point. (Recently a new airstrip was put in right beside the homestead which now saves considerable time when flying.)

It was going to be a full day and I would need it all. I also wanted to be back before dark. I have flown home in the dark before but without instruments it is no fun — nor is landing on the unlit Omaka airfield. So I had to be finished at least an hour before the darkness fell, leaving time to get back to the plane as well. At dawn I rang Shayne at Waitai for a weather update and at that time all was peaceful. No wind. I grabbed a quick cup of tea and breakfast and drove to my hangar at Omaka on the outskirts of Blenheim where the Pawnee was waiting, all loaded up the previous evening. So it was over an hour later when I approached D'Urville at about 1500 feet. While the sea looked calm enough I could tell that there were a few ripples on the surface indicating some breeze from the nor'west. Should be OK though. Shayne was waiting at the top of the strip in the Toyota, having first cleared off a few sheep.

The Waitai airstrip is a short steep 300 metre strip running southeast along a ridge 500 feet above the beach of a small bay. It is a one-way strip with a high bank at the top end and once committed you can't abort the landing and 'go around' to have another try. I did my usual preliminary run a few feet above the strip to find that there was a significant tailwind and lift over the bottom edge.

Hindsight is great and I should have immediately made the decision to fly down to Greville Harbour and use the nicely sheltered, much easier strip there. However, that would have added two hours to the day as it would have taken Shayne an hour to get down there to pick me up and another hour back to Waitai Station. The day was already going to be a long one and there he was waiting.

I landed, but with the tailwind too fast, and bounced. Brakes don't work while airborne and as the plane floated along in the updraft the bank at the top end of the strip rapidly approached. A desperate situation called for drastic measures, and I drove the Pawnee onto the strip. We stayed there but unfortunately in the process chewed up the ground with the prop. Slightly shaken I parked on the small flat area at the top of the strip. Shayne wandered up and asked, 'Has your plane always had those curvy bits at the ends of the propeller?' The tips of the propeller blades had bent badly on hitting the ground. With a bent prop there was no way I would be flying home. It really was going to be a long day.

Shayne and Pam at the time had been managing Waitai Station for four or five years. I had seen and been a little involved in the improvement in the Romney flock and the performance of the Angus herd that had resulted from his management. Their daughter was also born during this period. And, as rural vets do, I got to know them well and enjoyed their friendship, often overnighting with them.

Shayne drove me in the Toyota along the farm track which ended in a steep drive down to the homestead and woolshed by the sea; the rams were here as well as the other animals I had to attend to. All work at Waitai was finished by midday and after lunch we headed back to the plane and tied it down and removed the prop. I wasn't too sure at this stage how I was going to get myself or it back to town but the prop was of little use where it was and in its current shape.

Gus Forgan met me at the airstrip in his reliable but rusty Toyota people-mover. (All things ferrous, including fence wires, quickly rust on the island, the result of salt-laden sea air.) Gus and Bex are a wonderful couple who have now been managing Patuki Station for 10 years. They arrived on the island shortly after their first daughter Lucy was born and the other two were born while they've been there. Bex was very much a city girl, a practising accountant with little understanding of the country before she arrived on D'Urville. They have both adapted well to the remote property where self-sufficiency is essential. The whole family has embraced the lifestyle. It is fascinating visiting them: Bex is always busy home-schooling the girls, gardening, milking the cow and helping Gus on the farm. Because of the difficulty getting things repaired Gus has had to work things out for himself. As well as being a very good farmer he has become a competent electrician, builder, mechanic and plumber. Apart from a lack of regular social contact theirs is a wonderful life, full of adventures for three vibrant young girls. The Forgan girls have become very independent and self-reliant and a delight to know. I wonder how long the family will stay on D'Urville Island. With secondary school education approaching, the far easier life of living closer to town might encourage them to leave, although I suspect it might take more than that to prise them away from this paradise.

Anyway, on the day of the propeller mishap, I imagined that I would probably be camping the night with them. That would be no hardship but more a pleasant occasion. But I learned that their fencer, who had been with them for the week, was heading home that evening and he would wait until I got through all the work and give me a lift back to town with him. It was too good an opportunity to miss because not only would he get me to the mainland in his boat but he would get me back to Blenheim that night. Getting a ride from French Pass to Blenheim was a godsend; that was going to be the really difficult bit and I might have had to wait several days for a lift. Steve and Janet would just have to wait.

So that was what happened. We did the rams and a couple of other jobs, shifting between each task on a four-wheel motorbike, and then sped to French Pass in the contractor's outboard. From there to Blenheim in his truck and three hours later, around 10 p.m., with the prop on my shoulder, I arrived home. In all I had spent the day using eight different modes of transport.

Two weeks later, on a beautifully calm morning, Ray Patchett flew me, the propeller and my son George back to D'Urville, where we put the now straight prop back on my Pawnee.

For some reason, although I really can't blame him, George flew back with Ray. While his Cessna 180 was a lot faster than the Pawnee I did pass them after half an hour because Ray was flying around doing steep turns up a side gully. He was showing George some of the intricacies of ag flying, and while George had always shown an interest in that type of flying after that experience he really was hooked. He is now a very experienced ag pilot in Gisborne and amazes me with his skills and ability in a very demanding flying job. Secretly I had also always wanted to be an ag pilot but knowing the attrition rate for the job in those days and knowing my nature I probably would not still be around.

So while my story had a happy ending it would, however, have all been very different if I had better assessed the dangers of landing on that strip that day. Andrew Whelan, a very experienced local ag pilot with an exemplary safety record, wouldn't have made the same mistake. Some weeks later on another trip to D'Urville Island to finally catch up with Steve and Janet at Ragged Point, I flew past Andrew who was spreading fertiliser on Paul Newton's property near Havelock. I wagged my wings and said a cheery 'Good morning, Andrew' over the radio.

'Where are you off to this beautiful morning?' he said.

'D'Urville.'

'Should be a good day for D'Urville.'

'I hope so — I don't like that Waitai strip in a nor'wester. It's not a nice place to be.'

'Oh no — it definitely is not!' he replied, and I could almost see him smiling.

While Andrew would have no doubt made a perfect landing under the same conditions he would more than likely have flown over, taken a look and wisely headed back to Blenheim.

WACKER – PJ

Wacker Anderson was a legend in Marlborough, long before I arrived in 1979.

A generation older than me, Wacker lived and sort of farmed at Mount Patriarch, at the end of the Northbank Road in the Wairau Valley, Marlborough's most substantial catchment.

We would occasionally be called to do something on his farm, TB testing cows or castrating a colt. More often Wacker would arrive in his genuine old London black cab to purchase something at the vet club, where I worked for three years when I first arrived in Blenheim.

He was a man of medium build with jet-black hair slicked back, and his swarthy skin had all the hallmarks of a heavy smoker. In short, Wacker looked like a bit of a rogue, and readers may recall Private Walker, the character in the TV show *Dad's Army*, who he closely resembled. Walker was always on the make. As was Wacker.

Legend had it that he'd been in the New Zealand Army in Italy during World War Two, where he engaged heavily in the black market. Petrol, cigarettes, food, army vehicles of all sorts, including tanks, and army stores were all traded with who knows whom. Wacker had returned after the war with a bulging bank account, however he'd achieved it, and bought Mount Patriarch, a pretty tough place in the shadow of the rugged Richmond Range. The flats were fertile but unmaintained and the hill country was rapidly reverting to scrub when I first visited. A few rangy cattle and some ragged-looking sheep grazed quietly about the flats.

In Blenheim, Wacker was famous for his past, but he'd done a few dodgy deals in town too. He was particularly famous for raffling the same Christmas turkey around numerous pubs. He and his mate would travel from pub to pub in the old London cab, selling a two bob raffle for a turkey.

'Fifty tickets, to be drawn tonight.'

At each one he'd read out the winner, who just happened to be there at the time. It was Wacker's accomplice, unknown to the patrons, and he won it at each of at least 10 pubs.

It was probably small change to Wacker, but that was the man. If there was a bob to be made, he'd make it.

Like most rogues and conmen, Wacker had a gentle side. He really did love his animals, and he took in a lot of young men who had been either in prison or in trouble with the law. He would give them lodgings and a small stipend in exchange for work on the farm. And he might even get them to be his accomplice around the pubs.

When I arrived at work at the vet club one morning, I looked at the workbook. There was a very unusual entry: Mount Patriarch, vaccinate 15 cats.

Now most people brought their cat to the clinic for its annual, or more often triennial, cat flu and snuffles vaccine. We would examine the cat, check it was healthy, and give it a subcutaneous injection of the vaccine in the scruff, behind the neck. Most cats never know they've had it. But a vet visit is a stressful time for a cat. They don't like leaving home, travelling in a car, or meeting strange people, as a rule.

So to go to someone's home for multiple cats was a reasonable request. But 15 cats? At Mount Patriarch, 60 kilometres up an unsealed road? It was certainly novel, so I put my hand up for the job. I'd been to the farm before, and it was always an adventure to see Wacker.

I loaded up the rather small Ford van the vet club committee had decided was suitable for their new vet. (It wasn't. It was too small and light for rough country road, and I was very pleased after a year to hand it on when a new graduate arrived.) I took off up the valley to Renwick, along State Highway Six to the Wairau Bridge, then turned left up the valley once over the river.

The North Bank is very different from the rest of Marlborough. It's made up of a series of steep streams running out of the very rugged forested Richmond Range, which divides the Wairau catchment from the Pelorus to the north and west. It's a rough and magnificent range rising to Mount Richmond at over 1700 metres and is nowhere less than 1100. The underlying geology is schist and semi-schist, and when the forest cover is removed it's very erodible. In the nineteenth century the Richmond Range was the centre of major gold rushes, mostly on the Pelorus side, but some on the Wairau.

The North Bank, lying under all this, is shaded from the sun, particularly in winter, and the frosts are harder, the rainfall higher than the land to the south of the Wairau. Over 150 years it's proved to be a bad place for farming on the hills, just too tough, demanding and unproductive. So the hills are either reverting to native, or adorned with *Pinus radiata*, another issue. Forestry has stabilised the hills, but after harvest, that geology is susceptible to the effects of heavy rain. (Part of my life as a rural councillor, that is years after this story, has been to try to convince foresters to think more about environmentally friendly harvesting and planting methods.) The flats are better, but are now being rapidly covered in grapes.

However in 1980, the time we're discussing, the North Bank was a serious, if minor part of Marlborough's pastoral farming community.

As I sped up the winding unsealed road, past the bushed headlands and into each successive narrow side-plain of farming, I thought of the farmers and the gold miners of the past. I wondered and mused about the very tough pioneers who had trekked these valleys and made their harsh lifestyles here.

After Top Valley, the last of the series of side streams, the road became even rougher as it wound for 45 minutes up the tight steep bank, never far from the Wairau River. Eventually I broke out onto the rather scruffy plains under Mount Patriarch and before long the old homestead was in sight.

The day was a bit dismal, misty and grey. There were some nice cattle in a paddock by the homestead as I pulled into the yard. Wacker emerged from the house to greet me.

'Gidday, young man.' He was brusque but friendly. 'Grab your gear and come inside.' His brilliantined hair shone in its ebony blackness as he led me inside. 'Watch your head, mate,' he called as he went through the back door.

Hanging from a meat hook in the middle of the doorway at head height was a huge ox liver, quite fresh, and dripping blood onto the concrete floor. I eased my way past this curiosity and entered the kitchen.

A tough-looking young man sat at the table, and a multitude of cats roamed the old room.

'Shut the bloody door, mate. Don't want to let the cats out.' Wacker was slicing strips from the liver and placing them on a plate. The cats gathered. Feeding time.

And then I noticed there was something odd about the cats. Each one had a small neatly shaved patch on the back of its neck.

'Hygiene, mate,' said Wacker. 'Don't want them getting infections from the needle.' Using a safety razor he and his man had carefully shaved a 2 centimetre square patch from every cat, down to the skin. It was all very neat and tidy.

I've never seen that before or since. Wacker had learnt something from the army: neatness, order. And as Wacker and his mate brought the 15 cats to me, one at a time, and I carefully vaccinated each one under their watchful scrutiny, I mused what a rich and wonderful life I was exposed to in rural Marlborough.

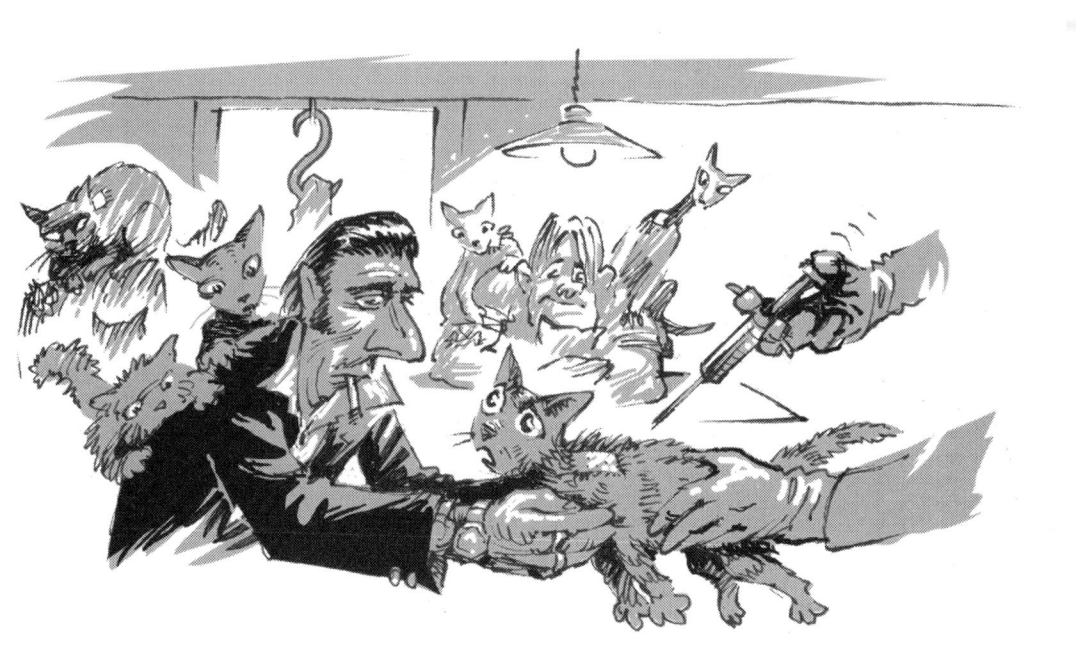

DRUG SHRINKAGE – PA

Deer had never really been farmed on a large scale anywhere in the world before we started it here in New Zealand in the early 1970s. As a result there was very little published information or knowledge about deer farming for any of us to fall back on. We had to learn alongside the farmers as we went, about all aspects of deer health and performance and how to manage them in captivity. We were also involved in one way or another with their capture. In the early days of deer farming, yards and sheds were often primitive affairs and any means of restraint like crushes non-existent so resorting to the dart gun was not uncommon. Using darts which are only capable of holding a small volume of liquid meant a small dose of tranquiliser had to be effective to heavily sedate a wild animal for capture or to remove the new season's antler growth from stags in captivity. We were suddenly introduced to a new range of potent tranquilisers, the demand for which we soon found exceeded our immediate requirements in the veterinary field. Others, including those capturing deer from helicopters, some deer farmers, and those wanting to experiment on themselves, were all desperate to get hold of these 'restricted' drugs.

As stags first start to grow their new season's antlers this rapidly developing tissue goes through a phase during which its surface has a soft velvety appearance. This unique, soft and very vascular tissue, known as 'velvet', is a valuable dietary supplement used extensively in Chinese medicine. Because of this value it is harvested at a critical time during the late spring and early summer period. The other reason for removing velvet at this stage is that if it is left on it is prone to damage and causes discomfort for the stag. This is not an uncommon occurrence when running large mobs of stags. The new season's developing antler is very sensitive and cannot be removed without anaesthetising the velvet. This is usually achieved by first tranquilising the stag and then injecting local anaesthetic around the base of the antler before removal.

So the drugs used for capture and for develveting were very powerful and under strict control, with only vets and specially licenced operators using dart guns, usually operating from helicopters, having legal access to them. This created a problem. As well as there being a bit of a black market among farmers and hunters for the drugs there was also a demand for them from drug users who obviously saw an opportunity for a whole new range of experiences. Self-administration must have been a wonderful hallucinatory experience in some cases while for others it would have been lethal. The result was a spate of burglaries around the country and even some recorded deaths of users of these stolen drugs.

One drug that the burglars for some reason seemed to target, or perhaps it was just because it was invariably kept with other restricted drugs, was Euthatal or as we commonly called it — 'purple death'. This is a high-strength pentobarbitone, coloured purple, but was in the early days primarily used at lower strengths as a long-acting intravenous anaesthetic. As its name suggests this drug is used for euthanasing animals and is an essential in the drug cabinets of all veterinary practices. I have no idea why anyone would want to play around with it. It has a horribly drawn-out recovery phase and I always felt for my patients when we used it as an anaesthetic for long procedures before gaseous anaesthesia became routine. There is a very fine line between knocking yourself out for a few hours of sleep and knocking yourself out forever.

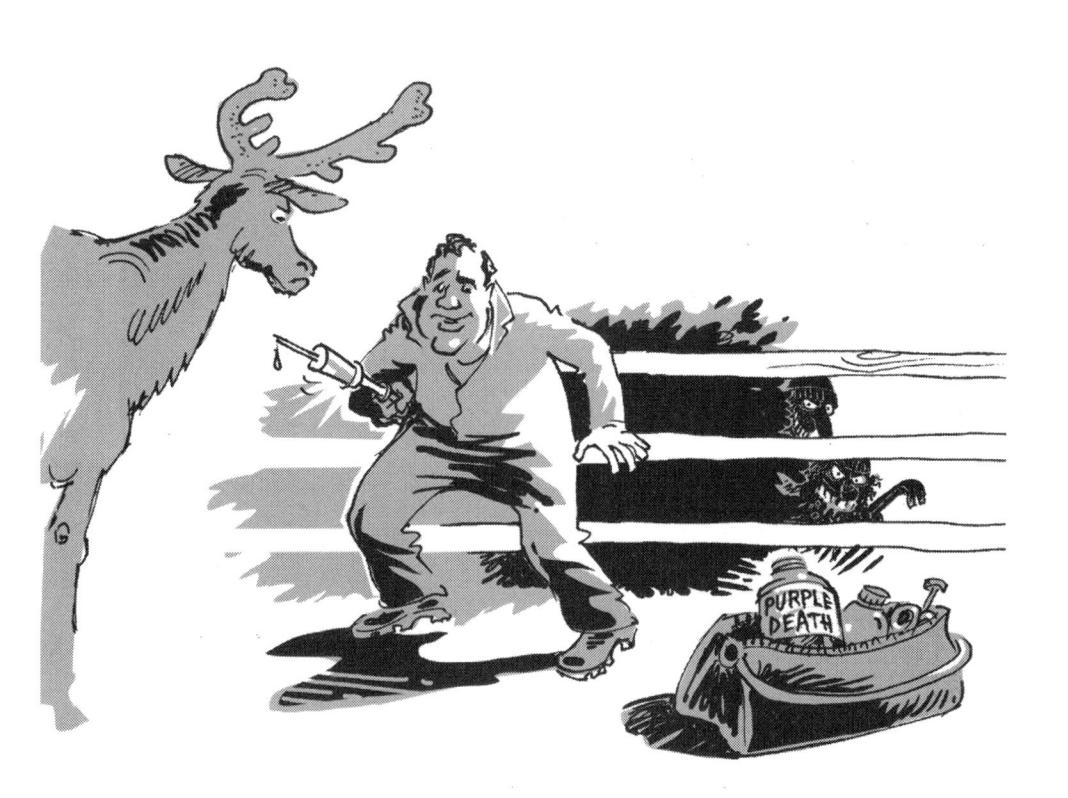

Some drug users did get their calculations wrong and went to sleep forever. In *Cock and Bull Stories* we tell how our clinic was broken into soon after Pete J and I set up on our own and several drugs (including our deer tranquilisers), two bottles of beer, and a dart gun were stolen. While the police did recover the dart gun it was not before a person had killed himself with the Anderson & Jerram clinic takings. It wasn't the pentobarbitone but a drug we used for inducing vomiting in dogs called Apomorphine. They obviously thought it was a sort of morphine and I suspect that person had a rather unpleasant death.

Another time my car was broken into while I was away with the family for a weekend. We found this a little disconcerting, suspecting our house had been watched and that they knew my car would have held drugs. On returning home and opening the garage door I found the boot jemmied open and all the drugs from inside laid out on the garage floor. They had systematically gone through them all and taken the ones they wanted. These days we are far more careful about carrying such dangerous drugs in our vehicles. Only when they are known to be a likely requirement for a job do they make it to the car where they are by law placed in locked safes.

Luckily the era when practices needed to carry large quantities of high-potency deer capture drugs has also passed. As the economics of deer farming have become more marginal, and the number of farmed deer is more than enough to provide replacements, the value of wild captured animals has plummeted and there is not the same demand for these drugs. No doubt word has spread throughout the underworld that the returns from breaking into veterinary practices are not worth the hassle.

In those early days, Noel McGirr, a North Canterbury vet, good friend and real character with a wonderful sense of humour, tells of the time he arrived at his Amberley clinic one morning to find the back window jemmied open. On cautiously entering the clinic through the rear entrance he could hear what sounded like one of the kennelled dogs groaning. However, he soon realised the groaning was not coming from the kennels but from the surgery. The first thing he noticed when peering into the surgery was that the drug cabinet was open. He then became aware of a very neatly dressed intruder lying on the floor below the cabinet from whence came the groaning. Beside him were two carry bags packed with a load of deer sedatives among old clothes and a tidy pair of shoes.

The intruder having found what he had come for obviously couldn't wait to try the product before leaving. He had already changed his clothes but hadn't got around to changing his shoes or making it to the door before the effects of the drug kicked in. While Noel waited for the police and ambulance to arrive he had an incoherent conversation with the robber. The latter did make some apologetic gestures to Noel as the police took him away and Noel believes he even promised reparation, but, not surprisingly, none was ever seen.

CONSUMMATE PROFESSIONALS — PJ

It's a strange old game, our one as vets. We're highly trained science-based professionals and mostly we earn the respect, and sometimes even the affection, of our many clients and often our patients too, especially the smaller ones.

Large animal vets are in an unusual situation when it comes to seeing our clients. We make house calls rather than our patients coming to us; most other professionals are visited in their offices, clinics or workplaces.

Being at our clients' farms means that we're slightly on the back foot. You have to tread very carefully on someone's home patch. On more than one occasion in my early career I was made to feel like the schoolboy visiting the headmaster by a couple of clients. While most of the farmers we saw were welcoming and generous, some were pretty standoffish, and one or two just damned rude. Many later became our lifelong friends, and it was very noticeable after Pete A and I set up our own private practice that the vast majority of our farmer clients did indeed become close to us. There was a respect for our being in private business, like them. The few who had been hard on us when we worked for the vet club generally stayed with the vet club.

These friendships meant that large animal work was rewarding and interesting and we looked forward to our farm calls. We would arrive and leave on the best of terms.

But just once I didn't. My professionalism slipped under some unusual stress factors, and I'm only slightly ashamed to admit I behaved inappropriately and lost a client. (Not that Graham was the only client we ever lost. We sacked a couple, who were just too hard to do business with, and in the big melting pot of human nature, a few probably didn't think we were good enough for them, for myriad reasons.)

The year 1989 was a horribly dry one in Marlborough. The south of this lovely region has a pretty dry climate anyway, but that year was a doozy. And when it's dry, farmers can struggle to feed their stock, and that understandably worries them. It can be very stressful. Their finances are often affected, and most farmers feel deeply for their animals. They hate seeing them suffer.

So that summer of 1989 and 1990 was a bad one. In March we were really busy pregnancy testing cows, with the empty ones going to the works to relieve the pressure on feed and to generate a bit of income.

Then Pete A crashed his aeroplane. He was flying in a very strong nor'wester, and had already had a big day when a gust tipped him as he was landing at Rod and Perena Heard's place at Kekerengu on the south coast. He landed upside down on a tennis court. The plane didn't bounce far from the point of impact.

Pete was badly injured, lucky to survive at all. His jaw and ribs were broken, his head badly lacerated, his skull cracked and he had very severe concussion. In truth, severe head injuries.

Pete and I had been Anderson & Jerram for about eight years at that stage. We were getting established, just raising our heads above financial waters, and we had a growing clientele. We were in our early forties, a very productive time of life, and we like to think we worked very hard. Our wives, Chick and Ally, would undoubtedly agree. They didn't see much of us.

There were still only the two of us, and it was getting to be a major juggling act to fit the large and small animal parts of our practice together. We would leave for work early, and come home late, nearly every day. With Pete out of action from his prang — he was in hospital for two or three weeks, then house-ridden for about three months — the pressure came heavily on yours truly.

I could see that I was going to have to get some help, and eventually I did when Mandy Batchelor, newly qualified, came and spent three months with me to ease the burden. (Mandy later came back and worked with us for some years and remains a good friend.)

But in the first three or four weeks I was pretty stretched.

When Graham rang, asking for his cows to be pregnancy tested on a day in April, two weeks away, I looked at the diary. Yes, I could do it that day, at 1 p.m.

'No,' said Graham, 'I want them done in the morning, so I can get them out the back in the afternoon.'

'I'm really sorry, Graham, but I've got a full clinic that morning. It'll have to be the afternoon.' I put down the phone, and gave the matter little more thought.

It had remained dry right into April. If you like summer living, Marlborough is a lovely place in autumns like that, but if you're a farmer, it's no fun at all during those years. And then, the day I was due to test Graham's cows, it rained. In fact it piddled down: soft, warm, life-giving rain.

My car, a Mitsubishi station wagon, was in hospital. It might have been because I'd driven it backwards into a telephone pole at 140 kilometres per hour, or it might have been for something more mundane, but whatever the reason, I had to borrow a car. The only one which Wadsco, the company we dealt with at the time, had available was a 1964 Holden Kingswood station wagon, an old dunger. It didn't look very professional, but it would do.

I raced through the clinic that morning, doing several small animal consultations, then some surgery.

I grabbed a sandwich, loaded my gear into the old car and headed up the road. Past Renwick I sped, then turned left into the Waihopai Valley road. These days the flats in the valley are clothed in grapevines, but in those days it was all dry land pastoral farming, and I ticked off the names of the farmers I knew well as I raced to Graham's place.

Over the Singing Bridge on the Waihopai River, and soon after I was there. I'd never been to Graham's farm before, and it was only later that I found out that Pete A had turned up there a month earlier to do the same job, only for Graham to realise he'd asked for March when he meant April.

The rain was coming steadily down as I went up the drive past the house. I could see the yards ahead and I was possibly driving a bit over enthusiastically as I approached. As I turned and braked, the wheels of the old Holden lost their grip on the greasy paddock, and the car did an undignified 20 metre skid before stopping more or less in the correct place. It was a spectacular but unseemly arrival.

I could see a pen full of cattle at the yards, a hundred metres away, and I could see two men sitting on a rail in the yards, unmoving. I thought my entry was pretty extraordinary, and funny too. I lifted the back door of the wagon and under its shelter donned my overalls and leggings, then took a handful of long gloves and a container of lubricant. One hundred and forty cows: this was going to be a breeze. The men sat watching.

As I trudged across to the yards in the steady soft rain, the two men still sat motionless, watching my approach. I climbed over the first pen and came up to them.

'Gidday, Graham, fantastic day.' I meant the rain was good.

Graham and his man were unmoved and his reply stunned and shocked me.

'No, it's not. I wanted you here this morning.' A hard, uncompromising glare came from my soon-to-be-no-longer client.

'Well, we're not going to let that spoil the day, are we?' I said, trying to be more cheerful than I was now feeling.

'It already has,' said Graham.

At that point, dear reader, something snapped in me.

I had been under near-unbearable pressure for weeks, with my partner and best mate badly injured. I had been juggling a lot of balls to keep the practice running, and I was probably getting a bit low on resources. Pete's accident had been front page news. Everyone knew he had had a very bad accident, and all our clients had been sympathetic, understanding and helpful. Until now.

I heard myself say, 'Well you might like to pregnancy test your own bloody cows,' as I abruptly about-turned. Seething but strangely exhilarated, I climbed the rail, stomped back to the car, whipped off my gear and jumped onto the old bench seat of the Holden.

I banged the column shift into first and planted the boot. A massive spin of the wheels and the rear end did a graceful pirouette, which turned into a full 360 degree wheelie before I headed for the gate. I should have been shocked and ashamed at my own rude behaviour, but I was almost ecstatic and the wheelie put the icing on it.

Something was released, and as I raced down the valley I found myself singing out loud — I felt as if I'd got out of jail free. The tensions of the last two months were gone. I'd been treated unreasonably, and had told my client so.

It wasn't very professional, but there's only so much a man can take.

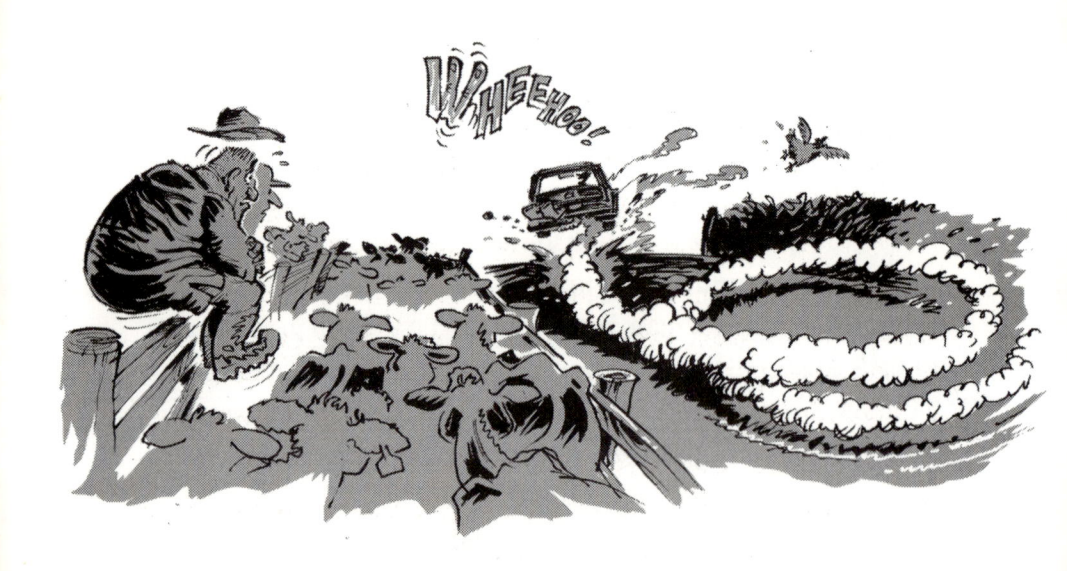

THE MULLER – PJ

The Marlborough high country figures prominently in my stories, and for that I make no apology.

That wonderful series of geographic features and the people who live and work there have long been where my heart lies. This love of the high country began when I spent early years working on large properties in northern Southland and Wanaka. The work ethic, the isolation, the tough thoughtful people, the self-reliance, the stock work, running and training dogs, and most of all the country itself, the beautiful surroundings, all capture the souls of the many people who experience it, and I am one of them.

Muller Station, next door to Molesworth at the head of the Awatere Valley, is one of the great high country runs, and I've been fortunate enough to have forged a lifetime friendship with the run holder, Steve Satterthwaite and his wife Mary. Together they run a very big station, one of the largest private properties in New Zealand.

My friendship with Steve began pretty early on, soon after my arrival in Marlborough. Paddy Dillon's cricket team, United Country, had established itself in my first summer, and in the subsequent winter I was in Christchurch for an international rugby game. I'd met Steve once or twice, so when we met in a bar after the game it was a natural gravitation. He talked of his love of cricket (although he hadn't played for 10 years since leaving school) so I suggested he should join our team. When the next season began he did, and quickly showed himself to be a punishing batsman, and not a bad medium-paced bowler.

That team became the focus of many family friendships, most of which have lasted, and after cricket Steve spent many evenings at our house in Blenheim, sometimes for a meal, sometimes for the night.

Steve and his family had had a disastrous and devastating year, losing two brothers to road accidents, and then his 10-month-old son to a cot death, all within three months, and I think Steve very much enjoyed the friendship on offer, and we became and remain good mates.

Steve's father Clive was a very successful businessman and farmer, and had set his sons up with farms, including Muller Station, which was run by a manager until Steve took over about 1978 or 1979. Clive was still pretty much a presence, a strong one, and we were a bit nervous around him. I recall him as an undemonstrative and firm man, but who knows what effect the loss of two sons and a grandson was having on him in the years I knew him.

He was rather stiff and unsmiling and I learned early on to tread carefully and to open my mouth only when I had something useful to say; despite opening the batting with me in a social cricket match in Canterbury, he remained pretty distant. The breakthrough came some years later when he came to Blenheim to watch Steve playing cricket. Steve and I had a long and productive partnership and, unusually, I scored at a faster clip than Steve. After that, Clive became much friendlier, and I felt I'd broken through.

The reason for his stiffness may have had something to do with an incident on the Awatere Road. Much earlier, probably two years after our first meeting, I was driving up that lonely winding path early one morning. I was off to perform artificial insemination on merino ewes at Glenlee, I think, or possibly to pregnancy test cows somewhere in the valley, and was approaching a small saddle, the Isis. It was a steep patch of road which had been tarsealed to consolidate the surface. Coming over the saddle and down the hill towards me was Steve's blue Falcon station wagon, no mistaking it.

As a back-country mate's gesture of friendship, I put my right arm out the window and vigorously gave the reverse victory sign, that is the fingers, to the approaching car. Sort of saying: 'Gidday, you old bastard.'

Horror! The impassive face of Clive, eyebrows slightly raised, slid past my window about a metre away, with Clive's lovely wife Diana looking strangely at me too. They had borrowed Steve's car. I'm sure the colour drained from my face as I planted the foot and raced on up the road.

I'd insulted the gaffer.

Over the years I did a lot of work at Muller Station, mostly pregnancy testing the 800-odd cows, and some deer work after Steve established a deer farm there. Steve and I became pretty good mates, and when his first marriage to Nicky dissolved and he was living alone, he spent many nights with our family in Blenheim. When his Jack Russell dog contracted TB, probably from catching ferrets on the station, it had to be euthanased and Steve was deeply affected by the loss of his little companion.

I also visited Molesworth with Steve, seeking high country brown trout on several occasions, often with Don Reid, Molesworth's manager. And when I received a business grant to travel internationally to learn more about dog cryogenetics (semen freezing) and transcervical insemination, Steve accompanied me across the western United States and up into Canada on a roadtrip. A highlight was coming out of Yellowstone National Park and staying in a motel run by an ex-F18 pilot who had flown 180 missions over North Vietnam, and also for Air America, the CIA's private air force, in Angola. Hayes Kirby was a character, and told us his story of being on a mission to 'take out' Idi Amin, the Ugandan dictator. The engines were running when the order to cancel the mission came through. We didn't doubt the truth of it. He had a lot of big photos of himself and his aeroplanes on the walls.

All the while, Steve was running the station with rare skill, with attention to detail and with real leadership, and he still does as I write this in 2016.

When he teamed up with Mary in the late 1990s he became a happier man again, and I was surprised and honoured when he asked me to be his best man. Mary particularly wanted a garden wedding beside a stream, so Ally and I were happy to offer our home on the banks of Spring Creek, near Blenheim, as the venue for the event.

Officiating at the wedding was John Craighead, a delightful man of the cloth who was semi-retired from that job, and mostly involved in his psychotherapy/counselling role. John is an old friend of my family so it was a pleasure to have him. He's relaxed and humorous, and it came as no surprise when he arrived and pulled out an old and rather grubby cassock, if that indeed is what the robe of an Anglican vicar is called.

It was autumn, and our neighbour across the creek was keen on the use of gas guns to scare birds off his grapes. In those days, Rapaura, heart of the grape country, could sound like the Balkans warzone that was a regular news item back then. This neighbour was particularly fond of his gas guns, and I'd rung him to ask if he could turn them off for a few hours while we had the wedding.

We set the scene with care. Straw bales were set out on the lawn for the 60 to 70 guests to sit on for the service. Steve and Mary's three-month-old baby Alice was tucked into her bassinet behind the large flax bush beside the pristine stream, which gurgled quietly and soothingly in the background. The happy couple stood, backs to the river, facing their seated friends. The Reverend, for that is what I feel I must call him for this story, raised his arms, spreading his slightly grubby robe for all to see, as he began the words of the wedding ceremony.

At that moment he was rudely interrupted.

Boom!...Boom!...Boom!

A trio of gas gun detonations rent the air. The neighbour, who shall go nameless, had either forgotten, ignored the message or, just possibly, was doing it deliberately.

Boom!...Boom!...Boom!

Gas guns make an extremely loud percussive noise, and you can't ignore them, or speak over them if they're close by.

After a few of these detonations, John Craighead remained undeterred. The show must go on despite the interference. He began to speak the words: 'We are gathered here...'

Boom!...Boom!...Boom!

Finally, with a broad smile, he made his greatest utterance.

'Well,' he said, 'I think I can say that this is the first proper shotgun wedding I've officiated at.'

Brilliant. The crowd dissolved in laughter and the show went on. And a jolly good show it was too.

THE LORD GOD MADE THEM ALL — PA

In *Cock and Bull Stories* I wrote about exotic animals and some of the difficulties vets are faced with when having to deal with them. My earliest experiences with a wide range of different species had been the animals at the Marlborough Zoological Gardens. This small wildlife park was developed in the early 1980s and survived for three or four years before a disaster and finances forced its closure. During the 1980s an influx of new species also arrived on the farming scene that presented us with many novel experiences and a huge range of opportunities.

There was a period in New Zealand's history when diversification in farming was being encouraged. It was not a big step to shift from sheep and beef cattle to include goats or deer in a farm business. After all they were both ruminants and there was some demand for their products: meat and fibre for goats, and meat and velvet for deer.

Both these industries have more or less successfully

continued in the New Zealand farming scene. Pete J in his chapter 'Angora Anguish' (page 47) tells of an interesting time doing embryo transfer work.

Many tried their hands at other species, historically not domestic animals, and while there are still a few around none have continued as a viable farming option. Among these were alpaca, Angora and rex rabbits, fitches (ferrets) and later ratites (emus and ostriches). The problem with this group was that once the initial demand for base stock was met — those that would be the nuclei for commercial populations — then there had to be a demand for their products either nationally or internationally in order for operators to survive. The message, well promoted by those people who were in right at the beginning, was that there was an insatiable demand for the products they produced — the skins and fibre from rabbits and fitches, fibre from alpaca, and oil and feathers and meat from ostriches and emus. So as well as the traditional sheep and beef and dairy farmers, many of those who got into 'farming' during this era were lifestyle-block holders, professionals and successful business people with money to invest. There was also an element involved who had somehow mysteriously acquired their wealth.

I worked with one rabbit farmer, Will Parsons. Rabbits were not the sort of diversification you would expect for a sheep and beef farmer, but he did appreciate their breeding potential well before he got into them. He was in right at the beginning and with the help of a regional development grant converted a hay barn into a purpose-built rabbit shed, and then imported 10 very valuable females and two bucks from Germany and set up a registered stud. By the time he had finished rabbit farming he was running around 800 Angora rabbits. As there were few other rabbit farmers in New Zealand to consult he had to learn much by trial and error. Breeding up was as expected not a problem, and feeding and management eventually, after some experimenting, became relatively easy, although fairly time consuming for a busy sheep farmer. Each rabbit was shorn four times per year and in a year produced up to 2.3 kilograms of very soft fine fibre. With an average value of $42 a kilogram the return from one little animal could be quite impressive. As a result, and being first off the block, there was much interest in his Angora rabbit farming enterprise. He once did a shearing demonstration in the wool room at the Ward A & P Show, packed to overflowing with punters including many local farmers. Merino farmers who had spent a lifetime having to deal with plagues of this rodent were amazed at the quantity and quality of fibre produced off such a small animal, but none could apparently identify with farming rabbits instead of merinos, even if it would have removed the concern of poor reproductive performance.

Will really enjoyed his rabbit farming days and paid a lot of attention to the rabbits' welfare and fed them well. Somewhat to his surprise he found that they had a very high pain threshold as they never flinched or reacted in any way if he happened to nick them during shearing. While shearing one particular doe he happened to nick it over a solid lump on its neck. He felt the lump needed further investigation so he carefully dissected out this large cyst-like mass from beneath the skin. He then stitched her up and made a special trip into town to show me this mysterious mass and see if I could determine what it was. He was a little taken aback when I began to laugh. I had to tell him he had chosen the wrong career and suggested he should seriously look at getting into cosmetic surgery. He had successfully removed a large lump of fat!

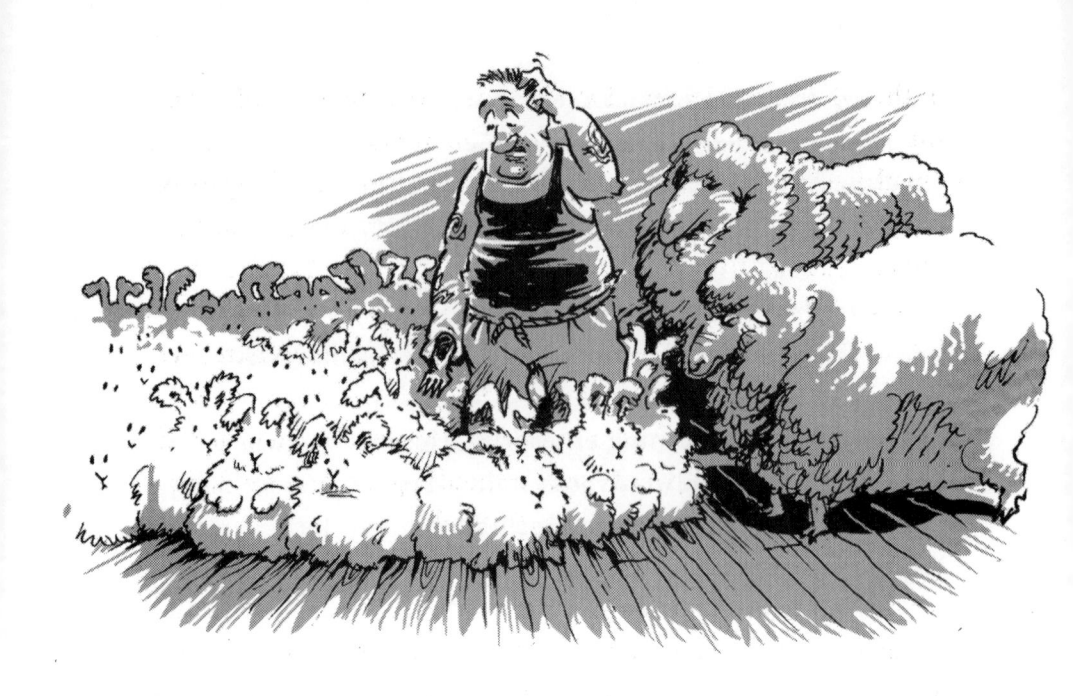

At its peak the rabbit fibre was worth $120 a kilogram. Will actually did very well out of selling the fibre as well as breeding animals for other budding rabbit farmers. The first doe he sold fetched $600. However, rabbits are extensively farmed in China and the Chinese quickly saw an opportunity to increase their Angora rabbit population. Within a year the return from the fibre started to fall and it was then that Will decided to get out. Luckily Robert Muldoon's livestock incentive scheme meant that Will did not lose too much when he sold, despite the value of fibre being a fraction of what it was when he bought in.

I was also involved with a fitch farm. These animals, ferrets, were bred for very high-quality pelts or skins and the group involved really went into it properly with a well-built house, cages and skin-processing equipment on top of very good management. Again success of this enterprise was determined by the value of the pelt and in their case the whims of fashion and the market. Within a couple of years the industry had collapsed. On the farm I was involved with, things were not helped by ringworm, a fungal skin disease, getting into the population. This disease ruined the pelts and was very difficult to control.

While I drew the line at ostriches and emus, Noel McGirr, our friend from North Canterbury, 'upskilled' in all matters related to ratite health and management. He went to several courses in New Zealand and overseas to learn about these birds so he would be in a position to help locals who wanted to get into the industry. I'm rather glad I left the ostriches to Noel.

The ostrich, native to Africa, had proved resilient in and adaptable to new environments and had been previously farmed in New Zealand on a small scale when ostrich feathers were a ladies fashion necessity. Emus are native to and farmed in Australia. A big new future was expected for these huge birds in the healthy red meat market, and for medicinal and cosmetic oils. Ostrich feathers, with their antistatic properties, were touted as the thing to dust your computer with. The unique eggs also had some novelty value. But I could never understand why anyone thought these birds would be an economic proposition in New Zealand if they were not flourishing industries in their native countries.

The ostrich is the largest living bird in the world with adults reaching 2 metres in height and weighing up to 150 kilograms. It is an extremely inquisitive bird and while quite intimidating when aroused, and capable of killing a lion with its big toe, it becomes reasonably docile when a bag is placed over its head. The emu on the other hand, while a smaller bird, is a real Aussie, being more fiery and difficult to subdue.

With the value of a breeding pair fetching $20,000–$30,000,

investment in the business was stimulated and opportunities were there for veterinarians. Fertile eggs were imported and sophisticated incubation technology implemented. Tricky surgical procedures involving risky anaesthesia became viable options, for example, to save valuable newly hatched chicks with retained yolk sacs, and to correct rotated and bent legs in older chicks using bone plates. Dealing with impacted intestines, the end result of their inquisitive nature, meaning they pecked at and swallowed anything shiny, was also not uncommon. Noel was kept busy with ostriches and emus for nearly 10 years, into the 1990s, but eventually the realisation that they were not going to live up to expectations forced most ratite farmers to cut their losses. However, Noel did learn a lot about a totally different type of animal, had some wonderful new experiences and also made many new friends.

We also worked with Peter Yealands, a well-known local entrepreneur now famous for his achievements in the wine industry. Among his numerous earlier ventures was deer farming, where Pete J and I were involved in carrying out embryo transfer work, and an attempt at possum farming. Peter felt that possum farming could be a viable option given, at the time, the value of the skins of wild-caught animals. However, success did depend on the skins being high-quality ones and that was influenced by time of year and the incidence of fighting wounds and skin damage. Peter felt that castrating the male possums would solve the fighting issues, so I had some interesting times sorting out an easy and economical way to anaesthetise and castrate them.

Again, as for fitches and rabbits, the market collapse spelled the end of that little venture. In Peter's case it was also not helped by a mass breakout from the enclosure where the possums were being held. Many of these beasts ended their lives shortly afterwards while mesmerised by the bright lights from fast approaching vehicles on the main trunkline and main road nearby.

Around about this time salmon farming had started in the Marlborough Sounds and I thought helping with the production and disease side of things would be an interesting sideline to get into. I was also advised that anyone with a veterinary background would be a useful addition to the local industry. As a result I spent a couple of weeks in Tasmania doing a course in marine farming at the aquaculture college in Launceston and returned an 'instant expert'. Unfortunately my credentials, to my surprise, didn't seem to impress either of the two local salmon farming companies. At the time both companies were desperate to identify the cause of a condition called 'bloat' but despite my numerous requests to look at sick salmon and past laboratory results I never heard back. Even though I had only done a crash course in fish farming I am sure with my veterinary training I could have helped get to the bottom of the problem. In hindsight I suspect they didn't want someone from outside being involved.

It is rather ironic that some time after this my daughter Caroline, who as a child had always been interested in veterinary things and often enjoyed watching me at work, ended up doing an aquaculture degree at Launceston after finishing high school. She returned to get a job with one of the salmon farming companies in the Sounds and became very involved in the work which finally identified the cause of bloat as being a nutritional imbalance.

This period in the 1980s was a wonderfully exciting era. We rapidly learned about all the various features and behaviours of a number of very diverse species, as well as different diseases, and how best to manage their populations. We became really competent at using new anaesthetics and often performing very intricate surgical techniques. We also made contact with a much wider and interesting element of society from where many new friendships developed.

In the end we learned that for a species to become established as a viably farmed production animal in New Zealand it has to provide a product, usually food, that is in constant demand elsewhere in the world. Hoping to successfully farm an introduced species that is not successfully farmed overseas or whose success depends on the whims of fashion is most unlikely to be a winner.

But for now the sun has just gone down and the cooler evening air is drawing in. I've done enough for the day and shut down the computer. After giving the screen a dusting with my ostrich feather, I'll don my ferret-skin jacket and then sit down for an ostrich steak dinner — washed down with a Dog Point pinot.

THE BENCH CLASS — PJ

I've always envied dog triallists. As a young man I worked on hill and high country farms, but only long enough to get a great love for those places. I had my own dogs, but only a couple at a time. I did train two as pups, a handy dog and a huntaway, and they both became pretty useful, but dog trialling is the sharp end of this. You have to be skilled and patient, you must know the character and temperament of each dog, and you have to understand and be able to read on the day the sheep's behaviour.

In short, you must be a good stockman, and most dog triallists I know would be in that category. My time on farms was too short to become part of that elite group but I still enjoyed running a dog. They're a proud lot, these folks, and to be called a 'good dog man' by one of them is a privilege and a compliment.

My friend Tony Sheild was one of the biggest farmers in Marlborough when I arrived in the region. That is not to say he was a big man. He wasn't, topping five foot six if he really tried, but he did farm a very large enterprise at Bankhouse, on the west of the Waihopai River, shortly before it joins the Wairau. It is, or was, a very large property, with almost 4000 hectares of flat land, and Tony ran his substantial Corriedale flock and his 200 Angus cows in a dedicated, efficient and productive manner, on extensive but dry river terrace country. He was pretty gruff, and in those days didn't suffer fools; I realised early on that you had to have your wits about you when you were dealing with Tony Sheild.

One gentleman who sailed with me for a while was the grain agent for stock firm Pyne Gould Guinness in Blenheim, a man by the name of George. Tony had rung George with a very large grass seed order one evening. Unfortunately George, who might have had a few that night, completely forgot the order. Its value was several thousand dollars, and I don't think George had a lot to do with Bankhouse after that.

That was Tony. But Tony was fair and very straight, and once you had his confidence, you had it for life.

Both Pete A and I were fortunate enough to be in that category, and Tony was not only a very significant client, he was a good friend to us both. We attended his children's weddings and socialised and sailed with Tony and his lovely wife, Puddy.

Tony called me one day. 'I want to see you. Are you in today?' I was, and we arranged a time.

When he arrived, he came into the consulting room and I waited the customary five minutes while he told me his latest yarn, usually one he'd learned from his dog trial mates. Tony was a very eminent dog triallist. I don't think he ever won a National title, but he qualified for the Island and National finals many times, mostly with heading dogs I think. At the time he came to see me he was national president of the

New Zealand Sheep Dog Trial Association and he remained in that position for some years.

The hugely popular TV programme *A Dog's Show* was once held at Bankhouse, and it was highly interesting sitting in the director's bus while the show was being filmed, watching how the picture was moved from screen to screen by a very intense small staff as they edited the show live.

I digress. When Tony had finished his story he came to the point. 'I want you to judge the Bench Class at the Nationals next month.'

I gulped. 'What the hell is the Bench Class, Tony?'

'It's the pretty dogs, the best-looking dogs. The owners parade them round, you have to select the best one. It's a piece of weasel's to a dog man like you.'

I wasn't sure. How on earth was I, a rural vet, going to pick the best-looking dog in front of a couple of hundred grizzled dog triallists? But Tony, being Tony, didn't take no for an answer, and when he left he knew I'd be there.

I have to admit I sweated on this one for a month. There was a real chance of making a fool of myself, and as I was just breaking through in the field of frozen dog semen, I would have quite a few clients and potential clients in the crowd. I needed to have some mana. Making a clown of myself wouldn't help that.

I rang Tony several times to find out a bit more and also Ken White, a cricketing friend who had won a national title, and had represented New Zealand in the UK, and in a test match versus Australia. A dog test, not a cricket one. Ken had a few words of advice. 'Go on gut instinct,' he said sagely.

But when the day came, I was still a bit anxious. The trials that year, doubling as both the South Island and National finals, were at Meadowbank, a large hill country property belonging to the Grigg family. It was only 5 kilometres out of Blenheim, easy to access for the many competitors and their families.

The South Island champs were held first, and after three days of that, a select group ran off for the National finals on the last day. On finals day at lunchtime, the Bench Class was held. A large crowd gathered to watch.

There were about 20 entrants: those triallists who reckoned they had the best-looking dog. The first problem was that there was only one class, so heading dogs and huntaways, very different physical specimens, were all together.

As instructed by Tony, I first asked all the contestants to form a circle around the perimeter of the ring. I had a nervous look around. There were black and white dogs, black and tan dogs, ginger dogs, tan and white dogs, black dogs, a white dog with a black patch on one eye. There were heavy dogs and very fine slim dogs. There were smooth-coated dogs and beardie dogs. How on earth was I going to make a reasoned judgement on who had the best-looking dog?

And then there were the owners. There were burly youngish men with cowboy hats, old grizzled men with cloth caps and walking sticks, men with pork pie hats. There was my friend Ken White with his prized heading dog. And there was Wes.

Wes was and is the beloved wife of my friend Mick Ensor, a delightful man, whose wonderful way of dealing with his stutter has endeared him to many. Mick's way of dealing with his affliction is to laugh uproariously at himself. It is one of his many traits which have made him a much-loved character. He and Wes farmed in Marlborough, and shifted in the 1980s to Wairarapa for a more reliable rainfall to farm with. There were many stories about Mick and his stutter, but the best was told to me by another farmer.

Once when trying to introduce Steve Satterthwaite to another farmer, Mick began: 'This is S-S-S-S-S-Steve . . . Sa-Sa-Sa — Sa — Sa — Saaa — Saatter . . . fucking prick of a name!'

Wes is a beautiful, graceful woman, tall and slim, calm and smiling. Mick was probably the more serious dog triallist, but in Wes he had a very able accomplice, and for the Bench Class you could only say he had an unfair advantage.

Hand on heart, readers, I did my best to be impartial. I asked the entrants to walk quietly around the ring in a circle, and then quickly settled on the best six, by pointing to each of them in turn. I didn't see what happened to those who missed out, but in the beer tent afterwards no one attacked me.

So I was left with six fine-looking dogs, and two of them were led by friends of mine. I'd reckon that's a very tough call, in what can only be described as a subjective competition. I was aware of the large crowd watching, and I was aware of the keen scrutiny of Tony Sheild, prominent in the front row. He would be a harsh critic if I got it wrong.

I asked the remaining six to parade again. Then I stopped, and looked closely over each dog in turn, examining the conformation, the head carriage, the alertness of eye, and the general impression. It really was very difficult.

I deliberated for only a short while as the crowd murmured in anticipation, or possibly in amusement. Then I made my decision. I pointed to the fine huntaway, standing quietly beside its proud owner. The owner was Wes. She was delighted of course, and was more than happy to take home the trophy.

I received a lot of ribbing for that decision. One of the finalists was even a little sour. He reckoned he had the best-looking dog. And in the beer tent, more than one friendly triallist reckoned it was Wes who'd won, not the dog.

I'm still not sure myself, but I do know what Tony told me a few days later: 'You got it right. You're a good dog man.'

I took that compliment. It's good to have loyal friends. But Wes is very lovely.

FOOTNOTE

Tony Sheild died in 2008 after a long battle with prostate cancer. Marlborough is the worse for his absence. Ten years earlier, when he was first diagnosed with the condition, he came to tell me about his problem at our clinic. He didn't know then how long he had.

'You know what, Pete?' he said. 'I'm really sorry about all the people I've pissed off.'

There may have been a few he'd upset (who hasn't?), but it was a gracious touch from a gruff man.

DAMAGE AND DUNG — PA

There are a few facts about faeces that you no doubt already appreciate. The first is they have an odour, frequently unpleasant, the second is they have significant sticking power, and third, the more liquid versions have an uncanny capacity to ooze into all handy cracks and crevices and to remain there forever. As rural vets we tend to live in the presence and smell of the stuff, but sometimes even we find that we have had enough and wish for a less odoriferous lifestyle.

I was reminded of this when I was asked to drop off a young black and white heading dog pup, inappropriately named Rock, at a property I was flying to one afternoon. He had been in the clinic for several days recovering from a parvovirus infection. Rock was one of the lucky ones that had survived this horrible infection and had supposedly recovered. Unfortunately in my car on the way to the aerodrome I was suddenly assaulted with the obnoxious odour of parvo diarrhoea. The poor little fellow had had a bad accident which was now flowing off the edges of the paper lining the bottom of the cage and all over the rear seat. The dysentery resulting from a parvovirus infection has a very distinctive odour to it — a strong objectionable and sickly one that permeates the environment. The smell is almost diagnostic of the disease. Despite a good scrub of the seat next day that odour took months to disappear from the car. Oh how I craved the old familiar smell of my car back again, the one that all vets' cars have, unpleasant to many but not us.

But that wasn't the end of the saga. After I had placed the cleaned-up Rock on the back seat of the plane I was using that day, the Marlborough Aero Club's Piper Cub BPG, and had taken off for Graham Black's property in the Awatere Valley, I got the pong again. Looking behind me I could see him heaving and squirting all at the same time. The force of his vomiting was also inducing projectile diarrhoea, both emissions paying no attention to the paper carefully placed in the cage under him. There was nothing I could do but fly on.

As BPG was frequently used by a number of aero club pilots I was not a popular person around there for some time until the smell finally disappeared. I was even less popular when, a few months later, and probably just after the odour had finally disappeared, the much-loved aircraft blew over and was written off after a flight into the Sounds (see page 62).

One of the few negative aspects of flying to the job is landing on an airstrip or paddock where cows have just been grazing. This often happened when I flew to outback yards to pregnancy test cows. Flying, instead of driving for hours, saved a huge amount of time and invariably allowed me to visit two or three properties in the same day. Frequently the herds would have been mustered in the previous day and had spent the night camped and defecating in the paddocks where I was expected to land. So when the wheels ploughed through the piles of dung on landing, as well as taking off, they would flick up the offending material to cake the underside of the wings and fuselage. As it might be days, and I confess to weeks sometimes, before I got around to washing it off, the dung would be seriously caked on and take some shifting. It was not easy for a not-so-supple back to get under a low-wing plane. I hate to think how much drag the thick layer of faecal cake was also causing.

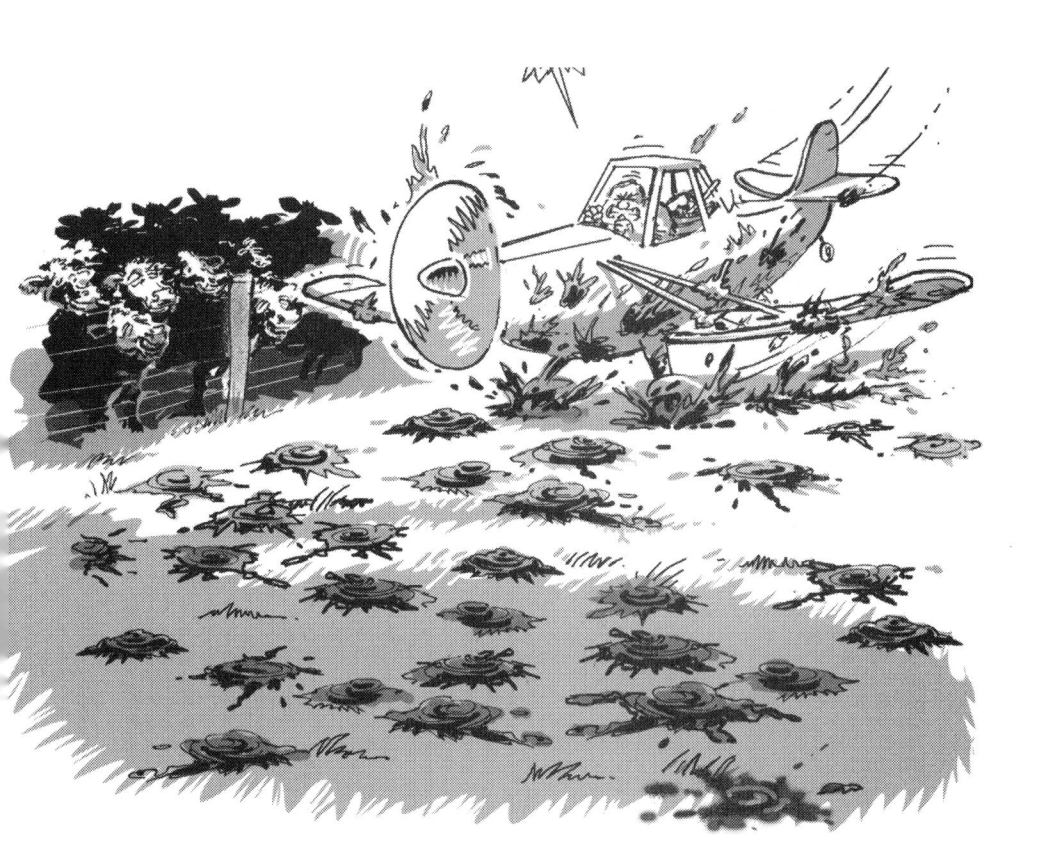

Dogs have been known to bring dung into my car as well, though not necessarily their own. Once I was calving a cow on a cold rainy early spring evening at Mahakipawa, a dairying area near Havelock. At the time I had a Holden station wagon, which I found to be a good rugged vehicle and useful on wet days because I could shelter under the rear door when organising gear for a job. On this occasion, when I lifted the rear door after arriving, the cattle dog thought the boot looked like a nice cosy place to shelter and keep warm, so in he leaped. In seconds he'd deposited an annoying quantity of wet dairy muck all over my surgical equipment, drug bottles and clean overalls. Detecting instant and obvious anger from me he leaped forward onto the back seat rather than jumping out past me. I raced around to get him out of there — and you guessed it he leaped forward onto the front seat. I managed to grab him and in the process of hauling him out he dragged with him my now soiled diary and the various papers that always lay on the front passenger seat. These fell into the mud and rain and became even more soiled. Unbelievably he thought it was all a fun game. The dog raced around the back and leaped in again. We repeated the whole sequence, all the while with Jarred Jenkins, the farmer, thinking it a great joke. I couldn't find anything to laugh about. My diary — an annual daily diary — was wet and muddy and would remain spoiled and tatty for the next four months. My diary is critical to how I work; as well as important telephone numbers, addresses and personal messages, it contains a daily to-do list and reminders of events in the future. I'm lost without it. Now I would be reminded of that bloody dog every day until the end of the year.

Then there was Roo, my old bull terrier, who used to travel with me a lot until one day he tried to walk on water. Well, dairy effluent actually. In the 1970s the standard of effluent disposal was not as good as it is now, and the wash often just accumulated in ponds next to the shed. These would with time develop a green growth on the surface, which to the uninitiated looked a little like a flat grassy area. However, if the surface was broken the contents underneath were usually black and sticky and very odoriferous.

I wasn't aware until I returned to the car that Roo had had a near-death experience. I used to let him wander around while I was working and when he got tired of looking for things to eat or play with he would return to the car and jump in the driver's window if I had left it open. The door bore witness to the fact that it was quite an effort for a bull terrier to jump up and pull himself through the window — the paintwork was well scratched. This time I could see the side of the door liberally smeared with black sludge and on looking in observed him curled up on my seat having made a half-hearted effort at cleaning himself on said seat and door and wherever he could find a bit of dry fabric. The stench that came out of the car was appalling although I sensed he was quite enjoying it. You could see where he had struggled across the effluent pond. He really was a miracle dog — walking on water... well, effluent.

Besides depositing faeces in or on vehicles, animals are also pretty good at damaging them. Every day when I get into my car I think of Charlie McLean's horse Ted, a friendly beast, who, while I was checking his foot, took a liking to the fabric of my door. I can now rest my arm in permanent deep gouges in the door or admire the chunks out of the rubber seal around the window, and am reminded of the day when Ted tried to eat my Holden.

I told the tale in *Cock and Bull Stories* about a sheep running to meet me on an airstrip on Malcolm Taylor's property in Ward, and tipping over my Piper Pawnee causing extensive damage to it as well as a little bit to myself. While a 70 kilogram animal could create a lot of grief for a 700 kilogram plane, a much smaller creature recently also contributed significant damage to the Pawnee. When I landed on a rough old lucerne paddock at Hunter Hills in the Hakataramea Valley, the tail wheel fell into the entrance to a rabbit burrow which caused it to snap off. Or perhaps it was a combination of an old crack in the tail wheel spring, a roughish strip and my technique.

One evening I was heading home from Mahakipawa, driving along the main road east towards Picton. It was the end of a long day and a pleasant evening, with the sun going down behind me. Ahead I could see a black and tan huntaway dog galloping along the middle of the road towards me. The dog was looking sideways into the paddock next to the road where Sid Mead, a local character and very keen dog trial man, was on his motorbike driving a group of heifers parallel to the road. Sid's dog was keeping a good eye on the heifers and as I slowed down I became aware that he probably hadn't yet seen me coming out of the setting sun. I slowed down further but still the dog kept up his steady onward pace, paying full attention to the heifers and little on where he was going. Eventually I stopped when I knew he definitely hadn't seen me. He smacked into the car doing a little damage to the grille but much more to himself. Sid Mead was very angry. His top trial dog had a badly broken leg and he didn't for one second believe that his prize huntaway had run into me and not me into his dog. I don't think he ever accepted that it wasn't my fault. I believe to appease him we repaired the leg at no cost.

Bigger animals can do even more damage. Over the years I had done quite a lot of work for James and Joy Jermyn. James has a wonderful dry sense of humour and Joy makes wonderful muffins. I always enjoyed the Jermyns' company and my visits to their farm. And James was usually prepared to give things a go if you could convince him of their value. This day we were testing his bulls for the first time to see if they passed a mating ability challenge.

As discussed in the chapter on bull testing, 'Veterinary Voyeurs' (page 163), the most important reason for a cow not getting in calf is the bull's inability to successfully mate with her. This may be due to a damaged penis, arthritis or poor libido. To test for the ability to mate we restrain a cow in a specially designed stall where the bull can mate her without too much stress on the cow. After we had set up the stall James wanted to move my ute and the trailer off the drive for some reason. I was a little uneasy because he wanted to place the ute in the large yard where the bulls were let out after testing. The sexual act can stir up testosterone levels and increase aggressive behaviour even in the most docile of males, but James assured me that the ute would be fine. His bulls were very quiet, he said.

After successfully passing their test, two bulls were let out into the yard, good mates until then, and got into a fine old scrap. The combined force of two bulls locked in combat is awe-inspiring. They become oblivious to anything that happens to be in their path — fences, gates, people and, in this instance, my ute. From my position on the rail I watched with mounting concern as these two gargantuan opponents wrestled their way around the yard. Accompanied by loud bellowing, and clouds of dust and stones flying in all directions, they bounced off the trunk of a large old gum tree, a post which made a loud cracking noise, and then my ute. It crumpled. Bonnet, front mudguard and driver's door all seriously caved in.

Another year in which I lost my no-claims bonus.

I don't get too emotionally involved with my vehicles but this was a smart new golden-coloured Holden ute which I actually quite liked. It was the same James who a few weeks earlier told me about the time he saw me arriving in the ute at a fundraising market day at Altimarloch, an Awatere Valley property. There was a good crowd there and I had my daughter Caroline with me. Anyway James was talking to a young lady there who was telling him she had just seen the most awesome car ever, a gold-coloured Holden with a really neat canopy. 'Gosh, it looked so cool,' she said. 'It just glided over the grass and pulled up beside us and then this really cool chick gets out of the passenger side.' And with obvious disappointment finished her story: 'But then this really old man falls out of the driver's side.'

Most rural vets do spend a lot of time in their vehicles and they are absolutely essential for the job. Sadly, but not surprisingly, a number of vets over the years have lost their lives in motor accidents. Tired, rushing to the next job, thinking about our last call or what we might be faced with at the next call can all distract us from the immediate driving job.

But to work as a large animal vet we have to get to where the animals are. The long hours in the vehicles, the distances, the terrain and the distractions, as well as the animals themselves, all conspire to have some impact on the state of our vehicles. We won't, however, call the insurance companies' attention to this fact.

ADMIRAL JERRAM — PJ

I think I've discussed my love of the sea in our first book. That love is deeply ingrained, from early days in dinghies at Waitati, north of Dunedin, where we had a crib, to sailing around the Marlborough Sounds and Cook Strait for several years. I even crewed with friends on a 44 foot yacht, *Vendetta*, on a 1700 mile trip from Hawaii to Tahiti in 1994, a wonderful experience.

There's also a bit of genealogy to blame. A perusal of our family history finds quite a few Royal Navy sailors, including two admirals. One of them was the stuff of legend, family legend that is, and our father told us many times of the famous Admiral Sir Martyn Jerram, hero of the Battle of Jutland in World War One. Hero in Dad's mind at least.

For the uninformed, Jutland was the only really major naval engagement of that sad conflict. The German Fleet, besieged in Kiev harbour by the Royal Navy for most of the war, ventured out into the North Sea. The subsequent battle was a bit of a stalemate, and although the Germans sank more ships, they never came out to fight again. A tactical draw, but a strategic victory for the RN.

I knew little about this as I grew up, just the name Jutland, and the family legend that our ancestor had made a big contribution to the battle.

So when I travelled up to the end of the Tetley Brook Road, south of Seddon, to Ian and Jenny Robertson's place, I was in for a surprise. Ian, a pleasant smiling farmer, about my age, greeted me in the yard.

'There's a bull with a crook foot and 80 cows to preg test, Pete.' It was my first few months in Marlborough and I hadn't been to Kainui, the Robertson farm before, and while I always like fresh country, you have to be on your game with new clients. I had a look at the bull, decided it was a developing infection, and gave it a big injection of Penstrep, the antibiotic combination most used then. After that the 80 cows didn't take long, and Ian and I yarned away as we worked.

'Come and have some lunch,' said Ian. 'Jenny's expecting you.'

It's a privilege to be asked into a farmer's house, and I rarely said no. One of our farm management lecturers at Lincoln College, Gerald Frengley, always said, 'Never turn down a cup of tea. You always learn a lot about the farmer' and he was right. The time inside, talking with a farming couple can reveal a huge amount about their aspirations, their understanding of their challenges, their attitudes to many things. I always enjoyed this part of the job, because the relationships PA and I had with our clients was hugely important to our business, but also to our lives in Marlborough. Many of these farmers became our good friends, the Robertsons among them.

I took off my overalls and boots at the car, donned my tidy clothes, and followed Ian inside. Jenny was preparing the lunch.

'Take Pete through to the other room, I won't be long,' she instructed Ian, and we moved into the sitting room. By the door was a large bookcase, and I could see at a glance that all the books were war histories. What a collection! I'd never seen such a good one, and although I've now got a substantial library myself, Ian's was a first for me.

Ian was pretty proud of it. 'My uncle left it to me. Help yourself to a look.'

I did and it didn't take long for my eyes to rest on a large heavy book, the spine of which had in bold letters 'JUTLAND, DECISIVE BATTLE'.

This was it! I knew nothing about the battle, but I knew about Admiral Sir Martyn Jerram.

'Could I have a look at this one?' I asked Ian.

'Of course,' he replied.

Excitedly I pulled the heavy volume from the bookcase, and thumbed my way through the index. Here it was! P384 . . . Jerram, Admiral Sir M.

With keen anticipation I found the page, and began to read. It went something like this:

At 1800 hours, Admiral Jerram's 2nd Battle Squadron sighted the masts of the enemy fleet. Signals were passed to Jerram's flagship, King George V, *that masts were in sight. An attack was urged by the sighting battleship at the rear of the squadron.*

Unsure as to whether it was friend or foe, and demonstrating a staggering lack of initiative, Jerram gave the order to the squadron to turn away and retire for the night. The decisive moment to win the battle was lost.

Horror! Trying to look nonchalant, so Ian wouldn't see my shock, I snapped the book shut, and pushed it back into its spot on the shelf.

'Find anything interesting?'

'Nah, nothing much. Good library though. I'm very envious.'

What a bummer. Thirty-two years of legend dashed.

There was nothing to do but head for the kitchen where lunch was ready.

TO CATCH A THIEF — PA

When I first started practising in Marlborough at the Graham Vet Club the cars were set up with radio-telephones (R/Ts). These were a very important means of communication, allowing us to keep in touch with the clinic and the other vets also out in the field. Directing to another call that might have just come in saved us much time and many kilometres of driving. R/Ts are still widely used in many practices although cell phones have superseded them in some areas, including ours.

In those early days the equipment was fairly primitive and prone to breaking down, in part possibly due to the shaking and dust they were exposed to along the many rough gravel roads we travelled. In Marlborough, with several farmed valleys lying between mountain ranges, reception could also be very poor. In those places we would stop at well-known spots where we knew we could 'get through' and actually understand what the other person was trying to tell us without countless requests to repeat themselves. While the areas for good reception with cell phones may not be much better, at least a message can be left when calls go unanswered.

Back then we shared a common R/T channel with Marlborough Transport and a couple of other businesses, and the conversations could be quite interesting. None more so than this story from John Smart, my classmate and good friend from South Otago who appeared in 'Just Do It' (page 41).

A sheep vet all his life and well-known identity in Balclutha, John worked for Clutha Vets. The practice shared a common R/T channel with quite a few other businesses in the greater South Otago area including Rosebank Davies, the local ready-mix concrete supplier, Milton Taxis and Brocks Transport (later Nyhons Transport) in Kaitangata. Nowadays most businesses have their own private R/T channel but in those days there were no secrets — everybody within earshot could hear what anybody on the channel was saying. This was at times a source of some entertainment and the practice being far and away the heaviest user of the R/T provided more than their fair share of amusing conversations.

In addition to the usual work matters — reporting on the completion of a call and receiving instructions on which farm to head to next — the R/T had other benefits. It was very useful for receiving updates on where traffic cops were hiding.

But the incident that John believes probably provided other users of the R/T channel with the most entertainment came one late spring day in 1988. The day had started off like any other and he had spent the morning out and about on farms doing his usual production animal work. When he got back to the clinic later in the morning the staff were in a bit of a flap. The clinic had been the victim of some shoplifting. It was in the fairly early days of Ivomec Injection, a newly released anthelmintic (wormer) for cattle which at the time was quite expensive at around $450–$500 for a 500 millilitre pack. We all had been made aware that a burglary ring interested in this product was operating throughout the country so most clinic staff were keeping an eye on things. John's staff were on the ball, had noticed the theft almost straight away and had the good sense to note down the vehicle details as the offender was driving off. Anyway, when John got back to the clinic Paul Winters, their merchandise manager, recounted the details — a scruffy-looking grey-haired bloke, unshaven, somewhat overweight, driving an early model dark green Mitsubishi Mirage, registration number such-and-such. The police had been duly notified.

John didn't think too much more about it until later that afternoon. He had calls 30 to 40 kilometres to the west of Balclutha into the Tuapeka Mouth, Clydevale area. After attending to a cattle beast at Ken and Allan Rishworth's and chatting about farming matters and having a pleasant lunch with them he headed back down the road towards Clydevale to the next call. John reckons that when he drove away that sunny afternoon in his comfortably warm vehicle he was in a very relaxed somnolent state and had to stop suddenly as he had slightly overshot the turn off to the next farm. Not only had he almost failed to turn right at the Clutha Valley School but he became conscious of the fact that there was a car approaching that he was meant to give way to. With the nose of his ute a foot or so across the centreline John, feeling slightly guilty, gave the driver an apologetic wave as he weaved past him.

As he turned and headed off towards Clydevale it slowly dawned on him that the other vehicle, and the driver at whom he had got a reasonable look as he negotiated his rather inappropriately positioned vehicle, possibly fitted the description of the thief at the clinic. By now well recovered from his dozy state he quickly did a U-turn and sped off after the green car. When he caught up with it he could confirm it was a Mitsubishi Mirage, but he could not remember the registration number so he called up the clinic on the R/T. Sure enough, it was the offending vehicle and, judging by the scruffy-looking driver, the same person. So for the next 30 minutes John followed this car around the district, giving Faye back in the office constant updates over the R/T about which road they were now turning into. Faye in turn was relaying this information to the police dispatcher, who in turn was passing the information by their R/T to the police car.

It didn't take long before the occupant of the car got a bit suspicious of the red Ford Falcon ute tailing him, speeding up and slowing down and following his erratic progress around the backblocks of South Otago. At one point, he pulled over and stopped on the side of the road in the middle of nowhere so John had no option but to do likewise and just sat in his ute behind him. The man finally got out of his car and approached John, who had the uneasy feeling that things could get a bit messy. He quietly locked the door. The man leaned down and through the slightly opened window, accused John of following him around, a not unreasonable accusation since this had by now been going on for at least half an hour. He then sloped back to his car and took off again. The description given to John by the clinic staff was pretty accurate. He was certainly unshaven, greying, overweight, a bit jowly and wearing old untidy clothes. Combined with being a total stranger he would have stood out like a sore thumb at the practice. It was little wonder the staff were immediately suspicious of him.

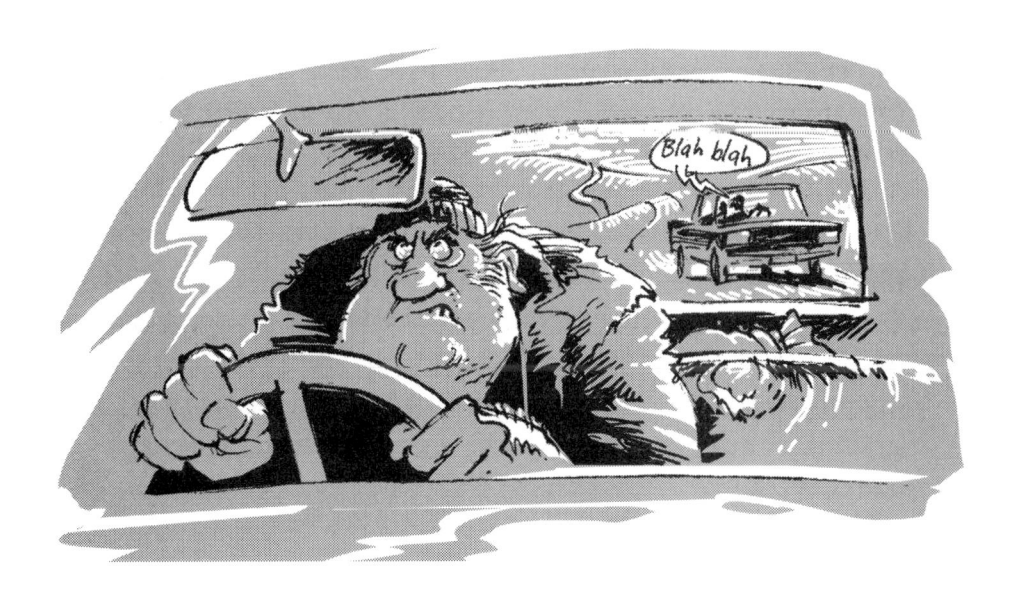

Obviously unfamiliar with the geography of the area he fortuitously headed back down the road towards Balclutha, in the direction from which the police would hopefully soon be coming. Very soon, from a high point on the road, John could see across a gully to a rapidly approaching police car maybe 2 to 3 kilometres in the distance, so he relayed their relative positions over the R/T and suggested he stop where he was and block the road. The unsuspecting thief came round a corner to find a police car in the middle of the road, and in a manoeuvre worthy of Starsky & Hutch, John boxed him in between the stationary police car and his vehicle. Lance Nicholas, the local constable, duly arrested the man and then, giving John a wink, suggested: 'Maybe you're in the wrong job, John.'

The thief turned out to be a fisherman from Featherston in the North Island who had been doing the rounds of veterinary clinics. Luckily Clutha Vet's Ivomec Injection was recovered in Balclutha from under a hedge where it had been dumped.

For some time afterwards John kept getting asked about his role in catching the thief, or had his leg pulled in some way by various locals who had either heard the transmissions directly or been told about the episode by someone who had. He was told that for some listening in to the R/T channel, work more or less ceased for the 30 to 40 minutes that the chase was on.

Usually unintentionally, we vets end up being the centre of entertainment and amusement, too often at our own expense. In John's case, however, he ended up a bit of a local celebrity.

And this time he really did have a good excuse for being late to his next call!

A HARD MAN – PJ

Halfway down the east coast of Marlborough, between Ward and Kekerengu, there is some beautiful fertile limestone-based hill country. It rises quite high to the majestic Benmore at 1244 metres, yet is close to the coast, and the views from the top are magnificent. It's good farming country too, and land down there stays in the same family for generations. The biggest river draining the country, the Ure or Waima, winds out of some pretty rough country in behind, then cuts through a long limestone gorge before emerging onto a flat riverbed notable for its white limestone gravel, as it meanders its last 8 or 9 kilometres to the sea.

It was late autumn on a cool morning as I turned onto the Ure Road off State Highway One, and cruised up the valley to Blue Mountain, the last property on the road. There are quite a few gates, I think I remember six which I had to open and shut, but at the last, there was the property owner, Dave Buick, opening it for me.

'Gidday, Dave, thanks for that.' I was truly grateful that he'd walked down the road to get the gate for me. Then, 'Hell, Dave, what've you done to your hand?'

It was wrapped in a very substantial bandage, with a couple of swollen fingers poking out the end. We had 150 cows to pregnancy test, and I wondered how Dave would work the head bail.

Dave looked embarrassed, but he gave a sheepish grin. 'Aw, the bloody hippy across the creek was coming over and bothering Lauren a bit, so I went over and fixed him up,' he confessed, then laughed. 'He won't do it again.' Lauren is a lovely, gentle and very attractive woman, and Dave was doing what most red-blooded husbands would do — protecting his patch. But I still wondered how he'd go in the cattle yards with one hand.

I shouldn't have worried. Dave is a tough guy, and as I worked my way through the cows, he barely flinched as he used his damaged hand. He'd spent years of his young life hunting deer for skins in the Canterbury high country, and a sore hand was just an inconvenience.

It had been a dry autumn and feed was short. Marlborough went through a prolonged drought in the 1980s lasting several years, and this was near the start of it, so farmers were pretty well stocked still. The upshot was, with feed short, Dave needed to get rid of some hungry mouths. I don't think he always preg tested his cows, but this year he was doing it to find the empties, so he could both lower the numbers and get a bit of cashflow.

It started with the first cow. Gloved and lubricated, I slipped my arm in, and immediately felt the foetus, bobbing in its sac of fluid.

'Pregnant,' I called.

'Bastard!' from Dave.

Next cow. 'Pregnant.'

'Bastard!'

And so it went for the next couple of hours. Normally farmers want as many cows as possible pregnant and are disappointed with every empty. A calf on the ground is money, and a cow which carries no calf has wasted a year of its productive life and eaten a lot of feed, for no net gain to the farming enterprise. But this time Dave wanted plenty of dry cows, and was looking forward to the cash. I think there were only two or three drys in the whole mob, and a constant refrain of 'Bastard' as I worked away, watching Dave's less-than-happy face with every call of 'Pregnant' I made.

At the end of the mob Dave was a bit cheesed off, but with typical hospitality he asked me up to the house for a meal, where Lauren cheered us both up with some nice lunch. I drove off down the valley later, reflecting on the wonderful range of personalities I came across in this fascinating job I had.

There's a bit of a postscript to this story.

Dave was a keen horseman, and either his or Lauren's favourite horse, named Donnington, a hunter I think, got pretty sick. Pete A was a much better horse vet than me, and he'd diagnosed an impacted caecum in the animal, which meant a reasonably severe colic, or a very sore tum. That's a crisis for a horse, one that takes some diagnosis, and one that many horses die from. It's the equivalent of appendicitis in a human, but the caecum is a very large organ, and horses are not the best patients for abdominal surgery.

The treatment for impacted caecum involves a laparotomy to extract the offending organ and surgically empty it. That's a major operation for country vets, bordering on heroic, but Pete was never short on accepting a challenge and he wanted to do it. Dave was pretty worried. He'd brought the horse into a paddock near Blenheim, and Pete asked me to come and do the anaesthetic. I had my old father staying with me, so I brought him along too. A retired medical specialist, he often came with me, and was always interested in the task and the people.

As I inserted the catheter into the jugular vein, then administered a litre of Glyceryl guaiacolate or 'GG', the horse's knees got a bit wobbly, and a couple of grams of Thiopentone sent it down gently on its side, deeply unconscious. (Younger vets will laugh at the anaesthetic mix, but that was what we had in those days, and we did OK with it.)

As the horse went down Dave cracked open a bottle of beer. 'Big bastard, isn't he?' he said cheerfully. Then, 'Like a beer, Doc?' to my father. It was about 1 p.m., so Dad declined.

Dave cheerfully sucked on that bottle, then another couple as Pete carefully prepared the abdomen, washed his own hands, gloved up and made his incisions.

Pete's a very skilful surgeon, and he made this difficult procedure look simple as he located the caecum in the very large tangle of abdominal contents. He was bang on in his diagnosis and as he eased the considerable mass of that organ, and quite a volume of large intestine as well, to the outside of the skin, Dave's vocabulary became more colourful, and more frequent. In fact it turned into a running commentary, punctuated with pretty rich language and the 'pop-clink' of bottle tops coming off. It was really very funny, but we were concentrating hard, Pete on his surgery — I gloved up and helped him empty the caecum for a while — and me on the anaesthetic.

I couldn't let Donnington wake up and I mustn't kill him, so doing all that made me feel, as always, that we had a few balls in the air. The long and the short of it is that Pete completed his surgery successfully and we felt quite pleased with ourselves.

We left with instructions for Dave and Lauren to roll the still-anaesthetised horse over every hour, until it woke.

As we drove away I asked my dad how he'd enjoyed the day.

He grinned. 'Colourful buggers, our farmers, aren't they?'

Yes, they are.

FOOTNOTE

Dave and Lauren told me years later how they had, as instructed, rolled the horse over every hour, until about four in the morning. Then they heard sounds of movement and found it standing. The horse lived, and hunted again. A moment of triumph for all.

TOOTED PACHYDERMS — PA

This is one of the best stories ever of a young vet being thrown in at the deep end. Picture a recent veterinary graduate fresh from university in his first job, alone except for a fellow classmate with even less experience, in a very remote part of the country. He is suddenly faced with a huge animal about which he knows absolutely nothing. Worse than that, this very valuable animal is afflicted with a condition for which there is no proven cure. The vet has a very limited arsenal of drugs and no idea whether the drugs he does have are sufficient in quantity or if they will work. And then to top it off he has not one but three crook monsters to deal with.

This is how a very young Vince Peterson, who soon after would become a well-known and much respected West Coast veterinarian, coped with a very difficult situation, totally outside of his comfort zone. Various versions of this story have appeared over the years but none of them by the person most intimately involved. It is best if Vince himself tells his story as it happened:

In 1964 when I was a new graduate the world was a vastly different environment to today. Many things which we now accept as part of the natural landscape didn't exist. All telephones were fixed to the wall with pre-dial handsets and they were operated through a manual exchange where the keyboard operators connected the calls as requested. Many of the drugs which we use today did not exist. Many of the surgical techniques we now accept without query had not been developed. Black and white television was just in its infancy and colour television hadn't yet been developed. And that was the world that existed when the circus arrived at Westport in the spring of that year.

For most of 1964 I had been the sole veterinarian on the entire West Coast since graduating at the start of that year. I had an area that I was responsible for which extended in the north to Seddonville, just south of Karamea on the Tasman coast, and eastwards to the Shenandoah Saddle on the road to Murchison at the top of the Maruia Valley. My territory went as far south as Paringa, a total area that stretched 240 kilometres north and 240 kilometres south. The Haast road opened in 1965.

In the spring, Dick Lim came to the Coast to work as a locum for a couple of months and he became part of what I now call the elephant story. Dick was a classmate of mine from our Sydney days and is Malaysian Chinese. He subsequently worked in New Zealand for several years then shifted to Australia and currently lives near Perth. Dick and I were at home in Hokitika one Sunday evening, which in itself was a rarity, when the phone rang. It was Joe, the owner of the circus which had just arrived in Westport, and he was in a panic.

'My elephants have eaten tutu and they are really crook.'

I explained to him that the native plant known as tutu produces a specific toxin for which there is no known antidote.

This is still as true now as it was back then. The symptoms in cattle include drooling, nausea, excitement, convulsions, coma and death. They may regurgitate as they cannot vomit. I told him that there would be little that I could do but he was adamant I had to come.

Dick and I had a discussion and decided that any attempts at treatment would be futile and, in addition, we did not have enough useful volume of drugs to attempt to medicate three elephants, each of which weighed in the proximity of 5 tonnes. We gathered what supplies we thought we may be able to use and set off north at full speed in my Volkswagen. The quickest route from Hokitika was through Greymouth then up the Coast road through Punakaiki then on to Westport, a run of about 160 kilometres. Dick hadn't been to Westport before and the state of the road north of Barrytown came as a shock to him. In those days it was unsealed, barely two car widths in parts and had many tight corners. By the time we arrived at Westport and pulled into the racecourse where the circus had set up its headquarters, Dick was feeling decidedly queasy and was several shades lighter than his normal skin colour. We soon found Joe and the elephants.

Apart from not knowing what is safe for them to eat, elephants are exceedingly clever animals. They were being transported around the country on a low-loader. This was not enclosed and contributed to what subsequently happened, as in those days the Upper Buller Gorge was narrow and unsealed. As the truck slowly wound its way down this road the elephants were helping themselves to anything they could reach. In the springtime tutu sends out long fronds and the elephants found these to their liking.

It was usual when they reached their destination that the

elephants unloaded themselves from their travelling platform, via four wooden half-barrel sections. The first three of these were laid down in a triangle with the base against the side of the truck, the fourth section fitting on top of the base. The elephants then stepped down using this construction. When they stepped down it became apparent immediately that things were far from right. Jodie, the baby at 21 years old and the cleverest of the three, collapsed and didn't move from where she had fallen. The two older females, Lena and Rill, were in the big top by the time we got there but were both obviously very unwell. Rill in particular kept going down and getting up again, accompanied by sounds of great pain.

The diagnosis was confirmed by the local boys who had gathered around to take in these strange sights. They had seen the tutu leaves that hadn't made it into the elephants' hungry mouths scattered over the decks of the truck and had announced with some certainty: 'Your elephants been tooted, mister.'

By the time we got there, a tarpaulin had been erected over Jodie out in the middle of the racetrack and an electric light had been set up so that we could see in what was now a dark night. Jodie was very unwell and every minute or so would convulse and stretch out her legs and neck with the familiar non-productive retching sounds of pain. A council of war followed while we figured out what could be done. It was Joe who decided that he had to talk to Lennie Larsen in Sydney, who provided the circus with veterinary advice when they were winter pastured near to Sydney. Professor Larsen had been my surgery lecturer little more than 12 months earlier and I thought that this would be a vain hope but if it gave some comfort to Joe, then that was what we would try to do.

Joe and I drove to the post office, leaving Dick in charge in our absence. We went up to the exchange switchboard and explained to one of the operators what we wanted to do. Somehow, and to this day it is a mystery to me how they did it, they tracked Prof Larsen down at his home in Sydney and he answered the call. Being Australian, the Prof knew nothing at all about tutu or tutu poisoning so he sidestepped the issue and said to Joe, 'Who is the vet you've got helping you?'

'Vince Peterson,' Joe said.

'You've got the right man for the job,' was Prof Larsen's reply as he hung up.

Good grief, if ever there was a hospital pass!

So it's all up to me and I knew nothing whatsoever about elephants, nothing of their anatomy, their physiology or anything.

Back at the big top Joe decided that we had to make the animals vomit. I tried to talk him out of it as they probably already had because of the nature of the tutu toxin and not only that, their internal organs had had enough stress and strain for one day. Joe wouldn't be dissuaded so off to town I went again after having phoned one of the local pharmacists who agreed to open up his shop late on a Sunday night. After the initial apologies for calling him out, I explained my predicament. Any emetics I may have had were designed for use in 20 kilogram dogs and that was a long way short of a 5 tonne elephant.

An examination of his apothecaries threw up one possibility and that was a chemical by the name of bismuth antimony tartrate which was known to cause vomiting in humans. I had never heard of it but the chemist said he thought he might have an old jar of it in his backroom of long-abandoned drugs. Sure enough he found one. It was an old-fashioned wide-mouthed ground glass jar with the corresponding stopper covered in years of dust. Once we had cleaned that off, it was time for some mathematics. Taking the dose for an average human weighing 80 kilograms and multiplying by 60 would be near enough. Once we had determined it could be administered intravenously, we made up three bottles of the drug dissolved in sterile saline and we were in business. Forget about the obvious errors of not knowing any inter-species dose rate differences, the obvious lack of sterility and lack of knowledge of anything whatsoever about elephant physiology; this would have to do.

Back at the big top I found that Dick had disappeared. While quizzing Joe about this, the mystery was suddenly resolved. One of the circus staff came running into the big top, his face as pale as Dick's had been some time earlier. He rushed up to Joe and said, 'Joe, Joe. I've just been out to check up on Jodie and there's a Chinaman out there leaning up against her and drinking a bottle of beer!'

Turned out that Dick had soon wearied of the aimless rushing around and had managed to find a bottle of beer as a replacement for the one that we had been looking forward to some hours earlier, before our abrupt departure for Westport. He had wandered out to where Jodie lay under her tarpaulin for a bit of peace. He found a convenient bale of hay which he pulled up behind her back and sat there contentedly while Jodie periodically went into her painful stretches.

In the big top I again explained to Joe that I preferred not to give the emetic but he wanted to try it on at least one elephant. Lena drew the short straw. She was the oldest and the biggest of the three and was the acknowledged leader. She was also the least affected by the tutu poison.

I was to find a vein at the back of one of her ears while the handler held her ear away from her body to give me access. Lena and Rill were both shackled to one of the big top's main poles but had limited movement which meant that standing beside a shoulder was possible. The idea was that the usual handler would pull the ear flap away from the body and I would stand alongside Lena while I inserted the needle into a vein.

What on earth?

I was wondering how multiple cuts over the back surface of Lena's ear had got there. Joe then told me that once the elephants were diagnosed as being poisoned by tutu, the 'locals' had advised him that the animals should be bled. What I was looking at was the result!

Until you stand beside an elephant, you don't have any idea of how big these animals are. Not only that but I knew that they had been falling down and getting up again, so it was with some trepidation that I stood alongside Lena. Thankfully she was as gentle as a lamb. It was easy to get a needle into a vein as they were at least 2 centimetres in diameter and having a needle inserted was probably a lot less painful than getting your ear slashed. Now I had to quickly attach the flutter valve, upend the bottle and get the solution in as fast as possible. Once the fluid was gone, I pulled the needle out and rapidly moved a comfortable distance away.

For what seemed like half a minute nothing happened, then Lena started to retch. She stretched out and extended her head and told the whole world that better things had happened to her. After about a minute the retching subsided and the spasms passed. The end result was that Lena's vomiting produced nothing. However, it did prove that intravenous bismuth antimony tartrate certainly causes vomiting in elephants.

I explained to Joe that they had all probably vomited as a result of the toxins they had eaten early on in the day and that it was probably not surprising that nothing further had been produced. With that in mind, thankfully the decision was made not to medicate the other two animals.

By now it was after midnight and we thought a cup of tea might be a good thing. One of the circus staff was sent to come back with a brew. We didn't have long to wait before the staff member returned with the news that there was no tea left in the circus. Joe then remembered that the 'locals' had also advised him that the poisoned animals should be drenched with cold tea. All the tea had been used to make the potion.

At this stage Joe told me that I had to get a 'needle' into Jodie's stomach to let out 'the gas' as she was the sickest of the three. This horrified me. Not only did I have no idea about elephant anatomy, but I was reasonably certain that gaseous distension was not a symptom of tutu poisoning. As well, the chance of putting a hole into a loop of bowel would almost certainly cause a fatal peritonitis — an infection of the abdominal lining and organs. However, Joe was determined that this must be done in order to try to save the animals.

Jodie was still lying down under the suspended tarpaulin. She was not happy and still spasmodically convulsing. I had with me a trocar and cannula: the cannula is a hollow metal sleeve about 1 centimetre in diameter and the trocar is the sharp cutting point that fits inside the sleeve. Once the trocar and cannula is inserted, the trocar can be withdrawn allowing any gas to be expelled through the hollow cannula. It works fine in cows that are suffering from bloat, but a poisoned elephant was something entirely different.

After the apparatus had been chemically disinfected it was time to give it a go. An elephant lying down comes nearly up to the top of the thighs when you stand behind it. The target was clearly undefined. All I could do was aim for the centre of the abdominal wall behind the rib area and hope for the best. Here goes! I grasped the instrument firmly in both hands, raised it up behind my head then with all my force I thrust down at the target. It was like hitting a trampoline. The trocar bounced back up almost to my eye level. I certainly felt the shock. Elephants, I found, have very thick and protective skin. The second time I managed to get the point of the trocar through the skin then, by twisting, I introduced it a further couple of centimetres, as far as I was game to go. I withdrew the central trocar and no gas came out the cannula.

At that point Joe appeared happy that there was no gas in there and I was certainly more than happy to stop what I was attempting. Surprisingly, it was easy to get an 18 gauge needle through the skin of Jodie's leg and I injected a 100 millilitre bottle of penicillin into her to complete the treatment.

Back in the big top, Rill had been getting up and lying down amid much obvious pain. Joe and the handlers decided they wanted to get Rill up and that they would use an innate habit of elephants to do so. Elephants try to lift others to their feet when they are cast and to this end they unshackled Lena to help Rill. The handler held the ankus, or stick that is used to control the elephants, over the top of her ear while the assistants unshackled Lena.

But Lena had had enough. Eating a plant that made her sick was bad enough but then being treated with a drug that made her vomit and feel terrible was the last straw. I will never forget the sight or the sound. She lifted her trunk up high and with a piercing trumpeting sound she charged away from where I was standing towards the end of the tent which rose up into the air as if it were a silk curtain. There was one more trumpet call from beyond the tent and Lena and her handler were gone; they had disappeared into the blackness of a Westport night.

We stood there shocked and stunned. Outside it was pitch black, and where do you go looking for a runaway elephant? Initially we could only wait, then after about 10 minutes the handler appeared through the end of the tent looking equally shocked. Lena had gone out the seaward entrance of the racecourse, then left into Derby Street and headed east at full pace. After about 100 metres she must have got annoyed with this weight tugging at the top of her ear for she suddenly stopped. Luckily for the handler he fell off as Lena cocked her trunk to the right then, with full force, lashed out to dislodge this annoyance to her left. She didn't hit the handler but she did lay two sheets of corrugated iron flat over the upper bearer of the fence that ran alongside the pavement to the rear of the main grandstand. Then she was gone again at full speed. The handler managed to see her heading across the road before she disappeared into the darkness. Lena was gone.

In the big top it was time for a tactical talk. Trying to find Lena would be nigh on impossible and even if she was found, in her mood and with the darkness, it would probably be difficult to handle her. Besides, Dick and I were conscious that we would have urgent calls to attend to in the morning. Talking to Joe, we decided that we could achieve nothing more there that night so we decided to head home to Hokitika. I arranged to talk to Joe the next morning to see how things had turned out. Driving through Westport at two in the morning was as quiet as would be expected in any New Zealand provincial town. It was a very dark night, with no light apart from the street lights, and nothing was moving. Somewhere not far away we knew there was an elephant on the loose.

When I spoke to Joe in the morning the news was much better. Lena had been found and recovered, Jodie was up on her feet although still suffering from a tutu hangover and the crisis was apparently over. It was obvious that the circus could not keep to its schedule as the elephants were not fit to travel, so the planned visits to Hokitika and Ross were cancelled and another day would be spent in Westport to let the elephants recuperate. I arranged to drive up to Westport on the Tuesday morning to check up on the animals and to confirm that they were on the mend.

On the Tuesday, Joe was much happier but still looking shell-shocked. The first story that came out was about Lena's recovery.

At dawn one of the locals who lived at the start of the Nine Mile Road got up at first light as per usual. It was spring and it was the whitebait season and Monty was going to chance his luck. He switched on the kettle and went out the back door to look at what the day promised. He glanced to the east of his back garden over towards the mouth of the Buller Gorge. The sky was just starting to pale and the stars starting to fade as he thought to himself that conditions looked just perfect for whitebaiting. He idly stretched as he looked around the section and he suddenly became aware in the gloom that there was an elephant in his vegetable garden, helping itself to his cabbages.

Momentarily stunned, he stood there until overcome with a sudden burst of energy, and ran back inside to tell his wife the news. She was less than impressed to be roused but reluctantly agreed to come and see if this wasn't a figment of his imagination. Lena proved to be cheerfully solid and Monty's wife was quick with the instructions.

'Ring the cops!'

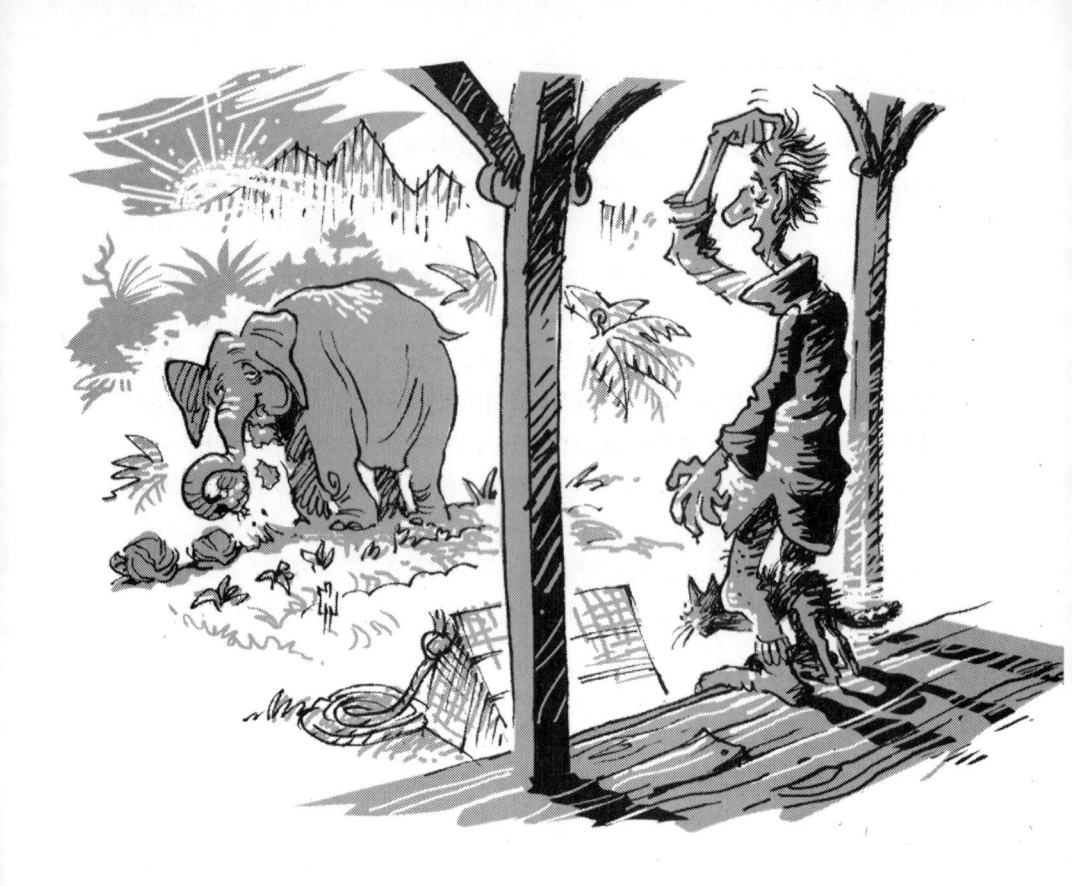

Monty did as he was told rather speedily. Westport in 1964 was typical of New Zealand provincial towns in that the police stations were manned throughout the night and Monty was soon talking to the duty constable. The response he got was gruff.

'Monty, I saw your car outside Digger's pub at about midnight. I think it would be a good idea if you went back to bed and forgot about whitebaiting for today.'

No amount of talk could convince the constable. He knew the circus was in town but the news of Lena's escape had obviously not reached the watch house. Luckily Monty knew the local police sergeant's home phone number and rang him. Once that conversation had occurred things happened in a hurry and it wasn't long before Lena was safely back at the circus, none the worse for wear, although you couldn't say the same for Monty's garden.

But Joe's story wasn't over yet. As he told it, by the time Monday night came he had been 48 hours without sleep and in a state of deep anxiety. For him, the elephants were the circus and without them his livelihood was mostly gone. What he needed now that the panic was over was a decent sleep. At least he could look forward to it knowing that his elephants were all apparently on the mend and not about to die. He and his wife were in their caravan preparing to go to bed.

They had a large van which had a separate bedroom at one end. Behind the bulkhead was a double wardrobe unit and when the tale unfolded, Joe's wife was standing behind the open door of the wardrobe which concealed her from anyone standing in the doorway. Joe was sitting on the edge of the double bed nearest the door feeling exhausted. That was the situation when a man walked in unannounced and asked to see the lion tamer.

As Joe retold it, such pranksters often appeared and were largely a nuisance that could be dissuaded with a bit of disarming conversation. Tonight Joe was in no mood for conversation but unknown to him this man, Ralph was his name, was cut from a different cloth. At first Joe replied that the lion tamer wasn't there but when Ralph became more insistent the exhausted Joe replied that he was the lion tamer and what did Ralph want?

Pulling out a large butcher's knife, Ralph raised it and took one step towards Joe with the words: 'Right, you're for it!'

What Ralph hadn't calculated on was that Joe's wife had heard the conversation, and from around the door she saw Ralph take a step forward. With that, she let out her loudest scream. In the small enclosed room it was deafening and Ralph dropped the knife, turned on his heels and bolted. By now Joe was wide awake and sleep was the last thing on his mind. In short order he was down at the watch house where he acquainted the duty constable with what had just happened.

'Don't worry about it,' said the constable, 'that will just be Ralph. We'll go and pick him up and see that he's looked after.'

As it transpired, Ralph was well known in Westport. He had a mental illness and outbursts such as this were apparently not uncommon and were usually resolved after a spell of treatment at the Seaview mental health unit in Hokitika.

Joe finally got his sleep but as he commented it had been a couple of eventful days.

By now it was obvious that the elephants were on the mend. Lena was none the worse for her emetic and subsequent escape and Jodie was back on her feet and the attempted trocarisation had not affected her. Joe decided they would stay until the next day and head for Greymouth and their one final West Coast appearance. I stressed to Joe that the elephants must make the longer trip through Reefton. Not only was the road wider with fewer bends but the elephants would not have the chance of getting into more tutu, which was a possibility on the narrow and twisty road through Punakaiki.

I headed home again thinking that I had finished dealing with the circus and their elephants. As it transpired that was wishful thinking. Mid-afternoon the next day there was a panic-stricken phone call from the circus saying to come straight away, that one of the elephants had fallen from their transporter near Mai Mai.

The road between Reefton and Greymouth roughly followed the railway line. There were several sharp crossings where the road, which ran parallel to the line, abruptly turned over it at right angles then turned as abruptly on the other side to continue on its way. This had been the cause of the accident. The elephants when travelling were shackled together at their ankles and held the tail of the one in front with their trunk. As they went, they rocked gently from side to side.

Rill was the unlucky one this time. She was still dozing, probably from the effects of the tutu toxin, and as she rocked gently from side to side the truck turned abruptly. When it turned sharply again on the other side of the railway line, Rill's sleepy sideways rock carried her over the edge of the deck and onto the road. She was dragged for several metres before the truck finally came to a halt. Luckily no serious damage was done but she had lost a fair bit of skin. I met the entourage near the Stillwater pub. I was pleased to see that the damage was thankfully superficial.

In those days we had a product called CT10 aerosol. It had two active ingredients, a now-banned antibiotic called Chloramphenicol and a purple antiseptic dye, gentian violet. It was widely used as a treatment for footrot in sheep until both ingredients were banned, the dye because it could not be scoured out of the wool. It also worked well on elephant skin abrasions and by the time the circus arrived at Greymouth, Rill had many bright purple patches down one side and on her legs.

I saw the two uninjured elephants perform that night in Greymouth and was particularly taken with Jodie who was obviously a very clever animal. So ended an eventful four days and this was my last contact with the circus.

There is a postscript to this story. Some years later a small news item in *The Press* caught my eye. It was headed 'Poisoned Circus Elephant Dies' and reported that a circus was camped near Brisbane and the elephants had been allowed to forage near their encampment. An elephant named Jodie had died after eating Cape tulip, which is a toxic Australian plant.

Jodie was smart, she was clever and she was a memorable creature. She had outlived her close encounter with tutu but another toxic plant had caused her demise. Such are the mysteries of life.

Looking back on this incident from the viewpoint of 50 years, three things have become clear under the sharp light of history. The first was the realisation of how little I knew as a recently graduated 23-year-old veterinarian. At least I tell myself I realised that back then. More to the point was the genuine affection that the circus owners and the rest of the staff had for their animals. They were a meal ticket but they were more than that, they were part of the family and the team had a duty of care to look after them and respect them. That was what they did in spades through large and small towns up and down the country. They were a travelling circus, but they were more than that, too. They had a unique way of life not experienced by anyone else.

What also is clear is that history has seen them swept away, gone in the inevitable process of advance, if that is what it is. No more will kids be able to experience the sights, sounds and smells of the circus animals. No more will they experience that anticipation of excitement and surprise. And no more will we ever hear again that voice of the eternal kid that lingers down through the years:

'Your elephants been tooted, mister.'

LIFE OR DEATH – PJ

'Old Thomas is crook, Pete. I think it's time to put him down.'

The words were depressingly familiar as I listened to the owner of the old dog. We stood in my consulting room in our nice new clinic, purpose built in Blenheim, and one we were pretty pleased with.

Thomas was an old bichon frise and his owners Alan and Sue Ellen were distraught.

'He can't see a bloody thing. I can't stand it,' said Alan. They were stoic but terribly distressed.

I knew Thomas pretty well. I'd looked after him for a long time, and had realised he was losing his eyesight. He had cataracts in both eyes, and although his cornea were both clear, the milky cloudiness of his lenses, and the wide-open irises, told the story.

'Is he eating?' I asked.

'Yes, but he bumps into things when we take him for a walk. It's not fair.' That was Sue Ellen.

'Does he mess inside?' Me.

'Hell no, he's too clean for that. He always goes outside.' Alan.

'Is he unhappy?' Me again, as I listened to his heart. It was slow and steady, no murmuring valves, no irregular rhythm. I listened to his lungs: clear and healthy. I felt his abdomen, and checked his lymph nodes. All clear. His gums were a healthy pink, and Thomas himself seemed unconcerned. Like most dogs he wasn't so keen to see the vet, but he was a cheerful little chap, and life was OK.

'So, he finds his way outside. What's he like in the garden?' I probed further.

'No problem there, he knows his way around.'

I knew this would be the answer. Many times I followed a similar line of questioning, and nine times out of ten, we came to the same conclusion.

'He doesn't need putting to sleep,' I said quietly. 'He's a healthy happy dog who can't see. But he's got a nose which can smell things that you and I wouldn't know about. He can find his way round home. Keep him there. He's got a few years in him yet.'

Alan and Sue Ellen were a bit doubtful, but obviously relieved. They'd come to the clinic, steeled and prepared for the worst. Now they were taking their little mate home again. They were good solid folk and I knew they would give Thomas every chance.

And they did. Years later, I ran into them in Bunnings where they both worked. Alan told me that Thomas had indeed remained a happy and contented dog for several years until his natural time came.

Euthanasing a dog or cat was something I could never do lightly. Some vets don't worry about it, but I always did, and like Alan and Sue Ellen, many owners really don't want to do it either. They just think they are doing their furry friend a favour.

Many times I've seen strong men and women, including farmers, completely heartbroken when I gave their old friend the lethal injection, sometimes sobbing uncontrollably. The truth is we build up a tremendous relationship with our animals, whether they're companions or working dogs. And because their lifespan is so much shorter than ours, we have to go through it time and again.

So I used to question most people pretty carefully when they made the appointment for a euthanasia. I'd like to think that over my career I might have given at least half of the doomed animals who came to me a longer life. In the majority of cases the owners were really grateful, but some were dubious, and a few downright angry. They didn't want to spend any more money on their pet, and who was I to tell them it wasn't necessary?

Well, tell that to a doctor, and while we as vets are fortunate to have the legal ability to euthanase, I never ever did it without a lot of thought, and often managed to change the client's mindset.

If the dog was still eating, not messing inside, still wagging its tail, let's look at this again. Sore leg? Let's see why.

If it's arthritis, we can help that.

Blind? Its nose is a wonderful and sensitive organ which lets the dog 'see' by smell.

And when it really was necessary, as I injected the lethal dose, and watched the animal gently close its eyes, I often found myself in tears with the family who loved their furry friend, or the farmer who was losing his best workmate.

I think I must be a soft bugger.

VETERINARY VOYEURS – PA

Working with farmers in a sheep and beef practice makes you very aware how important it is that all cows get in calf and get in calf early. As we've said one of our more important jobs has been to pregnancy test cows and identify their pregnancy status. For most of our careers Pete J and I did this manually and this job would occupy most of our day-to-day work from February until May. By the end of this period we were relatively fit but in my case I was a little bit off balance. Manual pregnancy testing involved putting on waterproof leggings and top and inserting a gloved and lubricated hand to the elbow or beyond up the cow's rectum. I mostly used my left arm for this and my right arm for holding the cow's tail and steadying myself and the cow, so different muscles were used by each arm. Surprisingly my right elbow these days is the one that seems to have the worst arthritis. As you can imagine doing the job over 1000 times in a day could be reasonably demanding. These days ultrasound scanning has made the job much easier but not nearly as warming.

How well the job went depended on the facilities, how wild the cows were and how much dry feed they had been on. While the faeces of cows that had been on dry rank pasture were not unpleasantly runny they could impede passage up the rectum and require raking out. Forgetting to bring gloves and lubricant could also make the job a little more difficult and unpleasant — as happened more than once with me when flying. After about 200 cows there were not too many hairs remaining on my left arm.

The two most common reasons for cows not getting in calf is either they are in poor condition, which often occurs after a hard winter, or they have not been successfully mated. Pregnancy testing time was usually when the farmer first knew that he had a problem and it was then that he also knew he wasn't going to be able to budget on a good return from his cows in a year's time. Depending on what we were finding as we were working, we might be in the presence of either a very happy farmer whose happiness improved, or one whose demeanour steadily deteriorated as the job progressed. At times like these I sometimes felt that the farmer was ready to shoot the messenger and I didn't enjoy having to mark each empty cow I found.

However, if the pregnancy rate was poor this was always a good opportunity to discuss with the farmer all the options and to start putting in place a plan to either find the cause or, if it was known, to implement management changes.

There are many reasons why a cow hasn't successfully mated or doesn't conceive. As a young vet I spent an inordinate amount of time when first faced with a problem farm looking for mineral and trace element deficiencies and certain diseases, but only occasionally found that one or other of these were contributing to poor in-calf rates. In the majority of cases the cause of poor reproductive performance in a beef herd was either that the mating cows were in very poor condition or that the bulls were not doing their job. So checking on the mating ability of bulls became an annual event on many farms, both to solve low pregnancy rates and to identify potential problems before they occurred.

We got into bull testing early on. While poor semen is often touted as a major cause of poor bull performance, in reality it is an insignificant reason. We did not waste too much time semen testing bulls as we were far more interested in wanting to know if the bulls were actually capable of doing their job, and we needed them to demonstrate to us that they could. This was carried out simply by restraining a quiet cow in a special stall or 'cradle' and watching the bulls mount her and achieve a successful mating. While smell is important for a bull to determine the time of oestrus in a cow, certain sights will also turn him on, just as with us men (PJ comment: PA is speaking for himself here!). All he needs is the rear view of a cow or the sight of another bull mating, or for that matter another cow riding a cow, to get him interested.

So we tested lots of run bulls — these being bulls of various ages on commercial farms. A herd of 200 cows might run six or seven bulls and we would test these fellows on an annual basis. Twenty to 30 per cent of bulls regularly failed the test. There were a number of reasons for failure including arthritis, penile defects and poor libido. In a study we carried out, just under 30 per cent of all bulls culled had become incapable because of arthritis, and most of these were not identified as having joint pain until they were put through the mating ability test. Trying to balance a couple of tonnes on one hind leg because the other one hurts means the mating procedure is very difficult and painful. Some bulls would not show any obvious signs of lameness until after an attempt or two at mating, observed while undergoing testing. It is easy to understand a bull's loss of enthusiasm for the job when he knows sex is going to hurt like hell.

A similar percentage of all bulls culled had defects of or damage to the penis. Most of these had developed after working for a season or two. The bulk of these penis problems definitely could not be picked up until we put them through the test. Nor could bulls with low libido be identified until tested. Some bulls — in our study 7 per cent of previously untested bulls — just don't want sex. Unfortunately because they never work they never wear out and invariably come in at the end of the season in great shape. On a number of occasions I have culled a bull because of low libido and the farmer has said, 'But he's my best bull.' No doubt because he had always held his condition while the rest had done all the work.

It is all very well for a stud breeder to guarantee a bull and replace one that doesn't perform, but lack of performance is usually not discovered until after the mating season and then you lose a whole year's production from all the cows the bull doesn't get in calf. As a result of our encouragement, and pressure from commercial beef breeders, our local stud farmers willingly got involved and had their young sale bulls tested. They appreciated that selling untested bulls was a bit like selling a new car without checking it had an engine, or at least one that started. A lack of libido is the most significant cause of underperformance by a two-year-old bull in his first season — so testing these bulls is important.

One stud farmer who was rather reluctant to submit his

young sale bulls to the test was Alistair Elliot, a most likeable character with many interests besides his Angus stud. He eventually realised he had to do it and on the afternoon of the test had called in his neighbour Andy Peter to help. Andy now owns this stud — but that has nothing to do with this story. This farm, at the bottom end of the Awatere Valley, has its cattle yards, where we were doing the job, right beside the Awatere Valley Road. Alistair was not really that enthused about the whole process and to begin with neither were his bulls. An initial lack of enthusiasm does sometimes happen when testing virgin bulls for the first time but when one eventually gets the idea the rest, except those with a low libido, happily follow. Alistair was probably beginning to think that perhaps he had a lot of low-libido bulls or that this mating ability test, or serving capacity test, or libido test, or whatever you want to call it, was of no use and we were wasting his time.

In the middle of this period of low activity a car pulled up and a well-dressed man with a cheerful disposition got out, wandered over and as is usually the case on such unplanned meetings remarked immediately about the wonderful weather before introducing himself. If he had been at all observant he would have noticed that little was bright and sunny over this set of cattle yards. Alistair grunted and then asked what he wanted.

It turned out he was selling fire extinguishers and opened his briefcase and pulled out a folder with all the varieties of extinguisher and the great deals his company had on offer. It was a very inappropriate thing to do. Alistair saw more than red fire extinguishers and ripped into the poor fellow.

'Can't you see we are extremely busy? The last thing I need right now is a bloody fire extinguisher and the last thing I want to do right now is to put out any bloody fire of any bloody sort.

Now get the hell out of it. Bugger off. Go away. Go. Go.'

By the end he was shouting and the fire extinguisher man rapidly retreated to his car and disappeared up the valley, no doubt hoping that the next farm he called at might be more welcoming.

Soon after this interlude the bulls started performing and the tension in the yards lifted. In no time we had done all 15 of them. All performed well except for one that had a persistent frenulum, a relatively rare event in a bull of this age. This is a band of tissue that extends from near the tip of the penis to the prepuce or sheath and prevents full extension of the penis. Normally this tissue breaks down at puberty. Alistair was delighted that I could fix it, which we did at the end of the day by simply snipping the tissue after tranquilising the bull.

The three of us sat down after all the work was finished, feeling at peace with the knowledge that it was a job well done with a good result.

'I'm converted,' said Alistair. 'All the bulls worked and you fixed the one that didn't.'

Andy and I had a good chuckle when Alistair then said, 'Oh dear, that poor fire extinguisher man. I guess I was a bit tough on him. Knowing my luck my house will burn down tonight.'

HELPING THE RAM OUT — PJ

I am the father of thousands of sheep, although I have never had emails or letters from my grateful offspring.

It's an unavoidable fact that most vet stories are about faeces, pus or sex. That's sort of what a rural vet's life is all about. This one's about sex, between sheep but with a human influence.

Prior to the mid-1980s the world of merino farmers was a pretty closed shop. The original genetics had been imported from Australia and the northern hemisphere many decades earlier. The Australian merino industry, much larger than ours, had a long-held policy of keeping their genetics to themselves, and New Zealand farmers had to make do with what genes we had in this country from those early days.

But sometime in the early 1980s that changed suddenly, with the breed association in Australia allowing the limited export of merino rams to New Zealand. The industry in both countries is a close one, and personal contacts between the two countries unlocked the door. Two things happened as a consequence. Rams were imported live to New Zealand and frozen semen was permitted to be imported.

While the first option, live rams, seemed the best bet, the practice quickly found a major stumbling block. Strict quarantine regulations in both countries, designed to keep a variety of pests and diseases out of New Zealand, meant rams had to spend several weeks in quarantine in Australia, prior to export. Unfortunately the Aussie requirements, or perhaps our own MAF ones, were that the ram had to be hard fed in the quarantine station. That means they were fed on dry pellets only, not green growing grass. From memory that was for somewhere between six and twelve weeks.

The consequence was that soon after arrival in New Zealand many rams were suddenly and disastrously affected with uroliths, or bladder stones. The problem was caused by minerals in the feed and the lack of a balanced diet in the absence of natural herbage.

A few Marlborough farmers were among the first to import Aussie rams, and several of them ran into trouble. Pete and I made a number of major surgical attempts to save these rams. The stones, about 2-3 millimetres in diameter, would form in the bladder then pass down the urethra. In the ram the urethra is a very long tube with a Z-shaped sigmoid flexure in the middle, and a fine tassel 2-3 centimetres long where it emerges from the tip of the penis. The tassel is designed to liberally spray the semen around in the ewe at mating to enhance the chance of sperm passing into the uterus. But the tassel is also a narrowing of the urethra, and many of the persistent uroliths would lodge there, preventing the ram from urinating.

These rams were often pretty crook by the time we saw

them, either on farm or brought into the clinic by the worried stud farmers. They'd spent a lot of money getting the rams here, and their future breeding programmes depended very much on the success of these animals. For most of these, and there were probably 10 or 15, if we couldn't massage it out, we would just snip off the tassel complete with stone. Most of the stones still in the bladder, or in the urethra, could then pass. The ram could then piddle and would recover quickly.

However, a couple had more serious blockages, further up the urethra, mostly around the zig-zag flexure in the middle of the ram's penis. These created a real problem. We would sedate or anaesthetise the ram to prevent spasms in the urethra, pass a catheter to the flexure, straighten that anatomical feature out by extending the penis, then try to flush the stones back up with pressurised fluid up the catheter. For some this worked, but we still had to remove the stones from the bladder, a significant operation in a ram. Full anaesthetic, incise the skin, then the abdominal midline, locate the bladder, incise into that, remove the stones (often many, like gravel) then suture the bladder so it was watertight and repair the abdominal wound. We would then watch the animal closely for several days, while keeping it on antibiotics, pain relief and muscle relaxants to help any remaining stones pass.

It was major stuff for the vets, the ram and of course for the farmer, who had invested a few thousand dollars on this ram.

On one occasion a ram was brought to the clinic by a worried farmer, a stud breeder. He left it with us, and we went to work. The stones were irretrievably stuck in the urethra, somewhere near the sigmoid flexure. We had it on the operating table in the clinic for a couple of hours and had cleared out the bladder, but we still couldn't get a catheter through the urethra, which is a pretty small tube. We rang the farmer, with Jill, our nurse, dialling the number and holding the phone to my ear.

'I'm sorry, Hamish, I just can't achieve this. It's beyond me.'

Hamish (not his real name) was not only unhappy, he was desperate and angry. He only just stopped short of calling both Pete A and me incompetent, and Pete said something pretty stern in reply. A vascular surgeon may have been able to cut and securely suture that very fine tube, but it was too much for us. Both Pete and I took pride in our work and thought we were good tidy surgeons, so it hurt a lot to be talked to like that, and Hamish was not only our client, but also our friend.

Sadly that ram was euthanased. Hamish was pretty upset at losing his investment, and we felt bad that we couldn't save the ram. But there was an upside. After many rams developed such problems the Aussies decided to allow the export of frozen semen from their sheep, and New Zealand merino farmers were to be the major recipients.

For me, the world changed about then. After a bit of a nudge from John Peter, a local farmer and Corriedale breeder, I made contact with a semen freezing and insemination centre in Albury Wodonga, on the New South Wales-Victoria border. I rang Neil Holt, the principal. Yes, he would train me, and a friend, for a not inconsiderable sum of money I might add.

I contacted my old university mate Richard Lee, a vet in Waipukurau. Would he like to learn to inseminate sheep with frozen semen? You bet he would. So in January 1986, Rick and I went to Albury. We had a fascinating week in the Riverina, spending days on large sheep stations learning to use the laparoscope, and more days in the clinic in Albury, collecting and freezing sheep semen.

There was a lot to learn in both disciplines. The laparoscope takes a while to get the hang of, co-ordinating hand and a refracted eye, at a distance of about 30 centimetres. The inseminating catheters they used were made from hollow glass tubing. They had to be made each night, prior to inseminating, over a Bunsen burner, drawing the melting tip out once, then again to a fine sharp point. It was laborious and exacting and by the time you'd made 200 or more it was bedtime. And the tips were very delicate. It was easy to break one off inside the ewe if she struggled in the cradle, or if you had to shift some inner fat to find the uterus. The joke was always that that lamb would be born with a glass eye, but it wasn't really funny at all. A piece of sharp glass inside a mammalian body can be very dangerous.

Freezing the semen was done by using an artificial vagina (AV), filled with warm water at body heat. A teaser ewe, brought to an artificial oestrous with oestrogen, was held in a cradle, rear end out. The collector knelt beside her, and the ram would approach, sometimes boldly, sometimes timidly, especially with a human so close.

When he mounted the ewe, you had to deftly deflect his penis with one hand and direct it into the AV, held in the other. If he was satisfied with that he would thrust and ejaculate immediately into the collecting vessel at the end of the AV. We would then quickly evaluate a drop of the semen under the microscope, estimate the sperm count, dilute it with egg yolk and store it in a warm water bath for the next step, chilling in a refrigerator. Then we froze it in a two-step process, first making pellets drop by drop onto a block of dry ice (carbon dioxide), then quickly tipping the pellets into liquid nitrogen for permanent storage.

The next few years meant pretty hectic autumns for me as the merino breeders, and those farming other breeds, took up the technology. It was a major change in our practice and it meant we eventually had to expand and hire another vet.

There was a lot to learn. I had to get familiar and competent with a difficult new technique. The fine hand-eye co-ordination required, and hours of concentration peering down a laparoscope literally gave me splitting headaches, particularly in the first year when I was aware of the importance of the outcome to the farmer and was finding the technique demanding.

Later I was a lot more relaxed as I became reasonably good at it. We also found some better catheters made of plastic with a fine needle tip, which could be sterilised and reused. Even better, they didn't break inside the ewe. This was a huge improvement.

We also had to learn about the vagaries of international shipping of hazardous goods; the semen is transported in special tanks containing liquid nitrogen, which at -270 degrees Centigrade can do a lot of harm if it gets loose. The bureaucracy around international freight was another large barrier, and there seemed to be little consistency between shipments. Many arrived only in the nick of time, and on one occasion at Blenheim Airport I almost had to physically threaten a deficient official at 7 a.m. I could see the tank through a doorway, but he told me opening time was 8 a.m. Meanwhile the ewes were ready and waiting an hour's drive away. I got the semen.

Preparing the ewes for artificial insemination (AI) was a serious, even critical part of the process. The farmer would select his ewes carefully for the genetics he wanted to enhance with a particular ram. They needed to be on a rising plane of nutrition so they would ovulate well, and then had to have their reproductive cycles synchronised so they all came in heat together, within a 24-hour period. Frozen semen has a pretty short life after thawing, as little as twelve hours, so catching the fertile eggs at the correct time is vital.

The ewes were synchronised with progesterone-impregnated sponges which were placed in their vaginas for 12 days then removed. At the same time as removal, they received an injection of follicle stimulating hormone (FSH) to increase the number of fertile eggs they would release. This improved the chances of one or more being fertilised.

So it all meant a lot of organisation, and the day of insemination was pre-ordained, weeks in advance.

I loved the whole process. It raised our precision standards, and got us very organised, but the contact with farmers was the great pleasure. They're good people, sheep farmers, and the merino breeders were, mostly, my friends, and still are. Spending a day in a woolshed with them while I worked intensively, and they brought the ewes to me one by one, was very satisfying.

The AI developments also led to a lot of similar work with red deer and wapiti, and with cashmere goats. Our veterinary world had expanded, very positively. Those years were the best of my professional life.

I took an assistant with me on the AI trips. Her job (I say 'her' because all the assistants happened to be women) was to thaw the semen, load the pipettes with the required dose, and direct them, one at a time, through the cannula into the ewe's abdomen. Peering through the laparoscope, I would then take over and deliver the semen into each horn of the uterus in turn.

The industry developed, and semen began to come in straws, not pellets. This required a different thawing regime. Bronwen Leonard was a very funny Glaswegian, whose husband Peter Orpin worked for us as a locum (see 'Beastly', page 223). Bronwen became my assistant for one season in the late 1980s. 'Blow, don't suck,' she would say sweetly as she thawed the straws into a glass tube, then giggled.

Sally Peter, another of my assistants for a season, was deeply concerned for the ewes, which had to be suspended upside down in front of me for the insemination. Some were clearly uncomfortable and would kick a bit, making my precision implanting very difficult.

Sally's solution was to take the stud book provided by the Australian company which supplied the ram and open it at the page with the photo of the ram we were using. She would place the open book upside down in front of the ewe's face, so she (the ewe) could see who she was being mated with. Sally claimed that the ewes were much more settled when she did this, and at least she (Sally) was happier.

Most of the young women who assisted me felt like that. They were empathetic and caring towards the animals, just as I was. I routinely used local anaesthetic on the puncture site of each ewe, and was very conscious that upside down, even though their bellies were empty after 24 hours in the yards, they could be profoundly uncomfortable. So the less time to perform the procedure the better.

The assistant's role was vital. It required the precision and gentle touch which women seem to inherently possess. The trouble was the assistants were all young and mostly married, and they all became pregnant in the same year as the sheep. I reckoned it was the pheromones from the AI job, but they didn't all agree. The upshot was that most seasons I had to train another assistant. Consequently there were often mistakes at the beginning of the season.

Jenny Jones, a hospital nurse, helped me with one of the early AI mobs at Richmond Brook, one of Marlborough's oldest and best-known properties.

John Macer, the manager, had befriended the owners of

Collinsville, a very large South Australian stud, and imported semen from them. It was the first time we'd inseminated at Richmond Brook, and the semen was very expensive, around $300 per pellet, which in 1986 was a lot of money. Every pellet was precious.

The day started well and by lunchtime I think we'd inseminated about 75 ewes, reasonable going at 25 per hour. I was being extra careful, and watching Jenny closely on her first day. She was quickly into the swing of it, neat and competent.

At lunchtime John was feeling pretty good, and probably relieved. 'Yvonne's got lunch at the house,' he said. Yvonne Richmond was a lovely person, thoughtful and interested, and she did indeed have a good lunch prepared.

The problem was Macer. He insisted on pulling out a cask of wine, and plying us all over lunch. Jenny had two glasses and I admit I felt a warm glow as we began again after the break.

Then, disaster.

'Oh hell,' wailed Jenny.

The first three pellets she'd pulled out of the nitrogen tank had slipped from her forceps, and dropped into the water bath as she tried to place them in the test tube. They were gone, no going back, $900 worth. There was a stunned silence, and poor Jenny felt terrible, but it was John's own fault, and he graciously admitted it, albeit through slightly gritted teeth.

But Jenny didn't ever offer to do the job again.

FOOTNOTE

The New Zealand merino industry made terrific strides in the following 20 years as farmers came to understand that better feeding of young stock meant a more productive ewe and would not affect the fineness of the wool. Coupled with new genetics as a result of AI, better feeding saw wool weights and lambing percentages increase significantly — just as many in the veterinary industry had predicted. It's fair to say that in the past, many farmers believed the solution to getting good fine wool was to keep feeding levels down.

That was a myth, and it also contributed to some pretty poor reproductive results. Lambing percentages in the 50s were not uncommon, and few achieved 100 per cent in those days. They do now, and Pete and I think we played a small part in this, both in our advocacy of growing bigger two-tooths and in our technical ability in AI. Does the industry see it that way? I hope so.

TRUCKING LIONS — PA

In the early 1980s a wildlife park was built near Renwick, a small town a few kilometres west of Blenheim. This was modelled very much along the lines of Orana Park in Christchurch. One of the principal initiators of the park was Murray Roberts who had been involved in the development of Orana Park and he became the first director of the Marlborough Zoological Park. After much fundraising and voluntary time spent building paddocks and shelters and enclosures, the animals had to be bought and collected.

I was involved with the development of the park and also the collection of some of the animals, a number of which came from Orana Park. We had bought two surplus lions, a tiger and a couple of water buffalo from Orana Park and they needed transporting up to Blenheim. The plan was to borrow a truck and go fetch them. The owner of the local wool store had kindly offered us an old truck they used for collecting wool from around the district. One Saturday I joined Mike McNulty, a member of the park's development committee who had a lot of experience driving trucks, and after a few issues getting the thing started we headed south.

Belching huge volumes of blue smoke, we headed up the Dashwood Pass, 10 kilometres south of Blenheim and arguably the worst stretch of State Highway One between Kaitaia and Bluff. At the top of the pass we came to the conclusion that this was going to be a painfully slow trip and from the smell and noise coming from the engine we were a little doubtful about getting to Christchurch and back, a round trip of around 600 kilometres. Being broken down on the side of the road with a tiger and two lions on the back would definitely have created a few issues, especially if it took some time for repairs to be carried out — that is if anyone was prepared to do repairs once they knew what we were transporting.

So we wisely returned to Blenheim. Luckily a good friend Murray Rose had kindly offered us his truck if we couldn't find another one, so after returning the first truck I phoned Murray whose immediate response was: 'Sure, and I'll come too. There's not much on this weekend and it should be good for a laugh.'

'Oh by the way I am out of miles and we can't get any more now,' he added. In those days a special licence was required to shift anything further than 50 miles by road. Trucks had a hubometer stuck to the wheels and miles had to be bought in advance.

'But I'm prepared to risk it,' he finished.

This was extremely generous of Murray because if we got caught he would be fined on several fronts: transporting on a Sunday, not having paid for miles, and not having a carrier licence and, I believe, transporting out of his area. Let's hope we didn't see any cops, or more importantly no cops saw us.

The three of us made it without any problems to Christchurch where we stayed the night before heading to Orana Park early on Sunday morning. Here we caught up with Murray Roberts and Orana Park's head keeper. There was a bit to do before we could load the animals — one was to vasectomise the male lion. Marlborough's park was only able to have a pair of lions as long as they didn't breed so we needed to see to the male.

That morning I could claim I had shot a tiger and two lions; something hunters pay a fortune to do these days. While I didn't have any trophies to mount on the wall, not that I would want them, I did have the satisfaction of seeing them quietly lying down and going to sleep after I had darted them. The tiger and lioness were gently placed into separate crates on the truck and given antidotes after which I vasectomised the lion, an interesting but relatively simple little surgical operation. I made sure I placed dissolving cat-gut sutures in his scrotum as I didn't fancy removing any sutures from any lion's scrotum in 10 days' time.

The buffaloes were reluctant travellers and it took some time to convince them that they should go up the ramp into their crates and join three serious predators on the back of the truck. We eventually succeeded and then made sure our precious cargo was safely strapped onto the deck. The load was covered with tarpaulins generously lent by New Zealand Railways.

Early in the afternoon we started for home. If all went well it was going to be at least a five hour trip. All did go well until just beyond Amberley, a town 35 kilometres north of Christchurch. The inevitable, and what we had hoped wouldn't happen, did happen. Mike noticed flashing red and blue lights in the rear vision mirror and pulled over. Bugger.

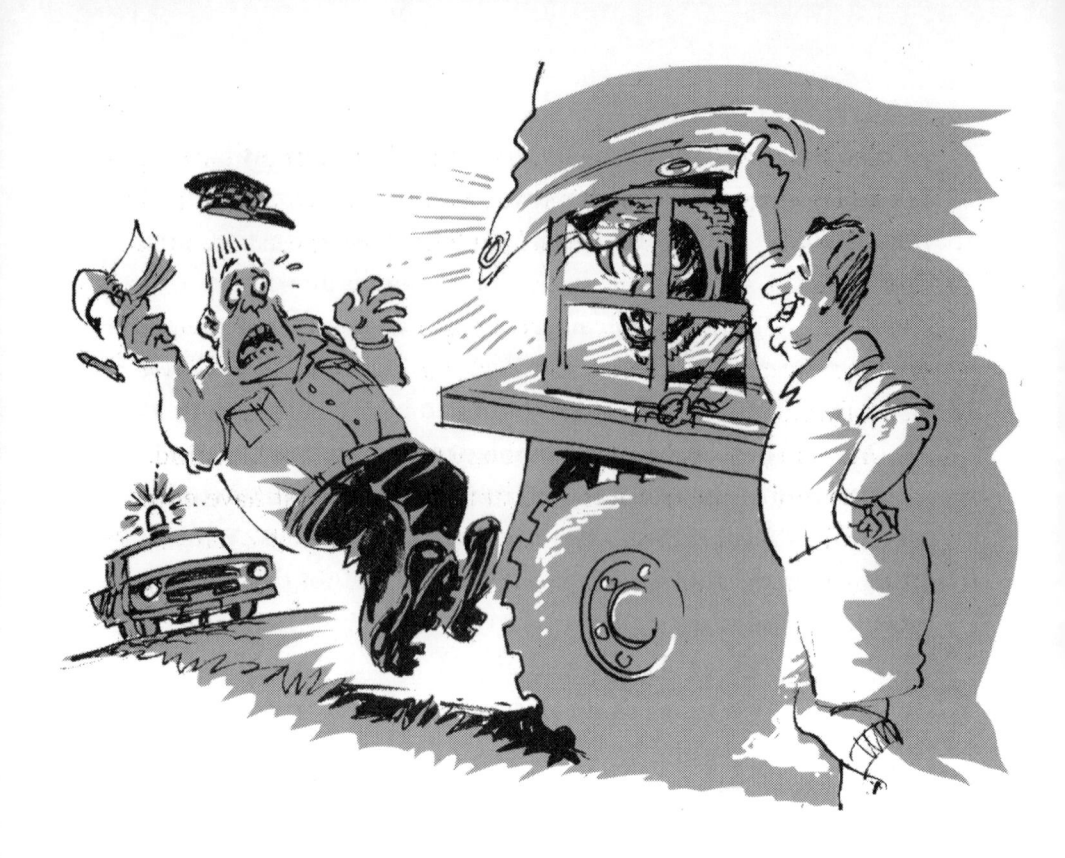

'You're a bit out of your territory. Where do you think you are going?' asked the traffic officer.

'Blenheim,' says Mike.

'And what are you carrying?'

'Lions and tigers,' says Murray.

'Oh yeah.' The cop wasn't impressed by what he thought was a very facetious reply.

By now I had had time to go around to the back of the truck and get between the cop and the hubometer. He turned and started moving towards me.

I lifted the bottom edge of the tarpaulin alongside the head of one of the large carnivores and told him to have a look. While the roar that came out of the small gap he was looking through startled me it must have given the traffic officer a mind-blowing fright. He staggered back, his ticket book flying in the air and, other than a very unprofessional expletive, was speechless for a moment.

When he had regained his composure he said, 'Well boys — you had better be on your way. You've a long way to go. Drive carefully. Go.'

All thoughts of checking a hubometer well out of his mind.

The rest of the trip was uneventful. Word must have gone up the line because on the way we were acknowledged and smiled at and waved to by at least two other traffic cops. He was a good cop.

EMBARRASSMENT AT THE BORDER — PJ

Fathering a lot of sheep was a very serious and important job, but it did have plenty of lighter moments. One of those came after my trip to Australia learning to freeze semen and to use the laparoscope to inseminate.

Rick Lee, my mate from Waipukurau, and I had about 10 days at Albury Wodonga, mostly apart, as Rick went off to the Riverina with one of the vets for on-farm inseminating, and I stayed at the centre learning to collect and freeze. Then we changed roles, and I had a wonderful three days near Jerilderie on one of the large polled merino studs. It was hard work, and while I was mostly the vet's assistant, I learned I had to concentrate very hard. It taught me to do the job for which I later had to train several assistants so the time spent was invaluable. It meant that I understood the job I was asking my assistant to do.

Every 15 or 20 ewes, Neil Holt, the principal of the facility, would say, 'Your turn to do the next three' and under his watchful eye, and the anxious scrutiny of the farmer, I would struggle my way through, handling the very fragile glass catheters that they used then to inseminate. I found the few I did each day to be really hard work. Back in Marlborough it took me a whole season before I felt really capable, and I could relax a little bit more as I did the job each autumn. But for several years, most nights I would come home with a headache, after six or eight hours peering hard down the 'scope.

When our time at Albury was finished, Rick and I bought some gear from the Holts. We didn't have artificial sheep vaginas at our practices in New Zealand, so we bought a couple each of those, and several of the latex liners and the glass collection vials that went with them. We embarked on a roadtrip back to Sydney, staying with a family friend in the Blue Mountains. A radiologist with a string of practices in NSW, David Badham was a delightful character, and his wife Bette a gracious and thoughtful host.

Dave put us on motorbikes to tour his rough bush farm, filled us full of beer and wine and let us know his thoughts on royalty in a very Australian way. When we learned it was Australia Day we started to sing 'God Save the Queen'. Dave leaped to his feet.

'Fuck the Bloody Queen!' he shouted, and stumped off to bed. (For years after whenever Rick was writing to me [before emails and the internet], he would put somewhere on the envelope, FTBQ, a reminder of that funny night.)

Coming back into Christchurch Airport I said to Rick, 'It's usually faster to declare we're vets and go through the MAF quarantine people. They're usually very good to vets.' So we did.

Ten minutes later I am standing in one of the two queues in quarantine, Rick slightly ahead of me in the other queue. There are a hundred people or more in the two lines. I watch as Rick is asked if he has anything to declare.

In a stentorian and very loud voice, loud enough for the whole concourse to hear, Rick says, 'YES, I HAVE AN ARTIFICIAL VAGINA!'

There was a shocked silence from the large crowd, every conversation stopped, and every eye turned towards the source of this statement, fascinated. The MAF officer, obviously embarrassed, could be seen leaning towards Rick and saying something, trying to hush him down.

'I SAID I'VE GOT AN ARTIFICIAL VAGINA!' he roared.

'Oh, that's what I thought you said,' muttered the inspector, puce with the attention of all upon him, and Rick was pushed rapidly out the exit door to freedom.

FAR FROM THE MADDING CROWD — PA

The earliest European settlers in Marlborough arrived by sea. With its sheltered waters, mild climate and plentiful supply of fish, the Marlborough Sounds became one of the first areas they inhabited. Although the terrain here and the natural fertility of the soil was not as suitable for farming as that of the Wairau plains or Awatere region, access to these areas from the south or from Nelson to the west was far more difficult. As a result much of these inland areas were bought by a few wealthier land acquirers, often absentee owners, who took over huge areas of the Marlborough countryside, while the smaller blocks in the Marlborough Sounds were settled by those escaping Britain, desperate for land of their own.

A sailing ship could drop off a family in any of the hundreds of bays where a temporary shelter could be quickly erected in the bush. Stores brought in and fish caught kept a man or family going while he cleared the surrounding native forest by axe and burning. Eventually most of the beautiful Sounds bush was gone, homes built and the land farmed. Burnt areas were hand-sown with English grass seed and pastures readily established on these cleared areas. A handful of cows and a few sheep and a horse or two were enough and the early Sounds farmers were soon in business. Good crops of barley and wheat, and oats for the horses, were grown on the flatter areas and most of these farming families were relatively self-sufficient.

By the middle of last century the fertility in the thin topsoil left after the bush had been cleared had all but gone. The cost of transporting stock and produce out and supplies in, either by long winding roads or by barge from Havelock or Picton, as well as getting expensive fertiliser onto the steep hills to maintain pasture production, made farming here uneconomic and forced many families off their land. Although one or two farmers on smaller properties stayed they did so by subsidising their main activity, milling the remnants of good native bush or by commercial fishing or later on mussel farming. However, most of the farms have been destocked and the land has reverted. The only areas still economic to farm lie in the easier country in the Kenepuru and the larger properties found in the outer Sounds.

When I arrived in Marlborough at the end of 1975 much of the land not farmed was either covered in gorse or in the early stages of being planted in pine forests. The gorse has been a wonderful nurse crop for the native forest to naturally regenerate and in some areas these hills must be getting back to how they would have looked when people first arrived here. Unfortunately the run-off from the pine forests, in particular after clearing, has become an environmental disaster. There are real fears for the long-term effects on the seabed and the water quality.

So what of the Sounds people? Their history and the environment have no doubt moulded them into what they are. Especially those who are descendants of the original farmers or those who have been working the land here for some time. As I've said farming really only continues these days in the Kenepuru Sound, which is off the main Pelorus Sound, and at the heads of both Queen Charlotte and Pelorus sounds and D'Urville Island. Driving to these areas takes time and steady nerves.

Farming the Sounds has resulted in a very self-reliant people. Needing someone to help with building or plumbing or electrical repairs or veterinary help is almost a sign of weakness. When you're asked to do some veterinary job in the Sounds it was often only because it was a dire emergency. But once there, all of these people treated us with wonderful hospitality and exceptional generosity. The pace of life appeared to be slower. In fact there was no merit in trying to hurry. These families became good friends and, once there, you didn't want to leave.

Colin and Mary Wells, Colin a descendant of Sounds boat builders and Mary of a pioneer Sounds farming family, bred ponies, goats, a rare breed of sheep — the Gotland Pelt — deer, alpacas, rabbits and Highland cattle. I often flew to their property in Nopera. Other than the odd emergency, such as a difficult calving, most work for them included the more routine develveting of stags and TB testing deer, or castrating colts. A visit to their well-lived-in house for a cup of tea was mandatory and usually only ended when rapidly failing daylight forced my departure. I always went home with a bucket of something, usually from the sea — oysters collected from the rocks earlier by Colin, or mussels from his mussel farm. He even encouraged me to dust off my golf clubs, unused since student days, and have a round of golf with him on the nine-hole Nopera golf course next to their property and the airstrip. These wonderful memories are saddened by my last recollection of Colin, who was dying from cancer, sitting in his truck joking away while watching his son Chris and I dehorn the 25 Highland cattle that were destined for the works. Because there was no decent race nor head-bail this job was proving somewhat difficult. I will always fondly remember this great Sounds couple and their family.

Margaret and David Harvey farmed in Beatrix Bay, off the outer Pelorus Sound. Margaret and her daughter Sally bred event-type hacks. Most work at the Harveys' was horse work and this particular day was no exception. A mare had foaled a couple of days earlier but still had a retained placenta. A retained placenta is serious if the mare cannot get rid of it within a few hours of foaling. A uterine infection and laminitis or 'founder' — inflammation of the laminae resulting in separation of the hoof from underlying bone — can set in and be fatal. Margaret knew this and wanted me out there 'reasonably soon' as the mare wasn't looking quite so perky. I flew to the neighbouring property where Margaret picked me up. As we drove to her place, she happened to mention, referring to the mare, that there seemed to be 'an awful lot of her hanging out'. Sure enough when we got there she was already starting to prolapse her uterus. Not a common event in a mare and potentially fatal. However, I managed to remove the placenta and replace the prolapsed uterus without too much difficulty.

I think the mare epitomised the Sounds people. While faced with a critical situation both she and Margaret remained calm which made my job so much easier. Dealing with nervous owners and excited patients always adds another dimension to our job. The Sounds residents who have spent their whole life there seem to have a relaxed and controlled and pragmatic approach to life.

Their kindness is another quality. When visiting Robin and Alison Bowron in Waitaria Bay I invariably left satiated in both mind and body. Alison is a great cook and also knows everything that is going on in the Sounds. I guess that is a spinoff from the days before the telephone and easier road access, when it was important that people knew what was happening at their neighbours. If anyone needed help it was going to come first from their closest neighbour — either via a horse track around the hills or across the bay by boat — so knowing what was happening next door was a survival thing. I usually came home from my visits to the Sounds with all the latest local news and gossip. The Bowrons had a very good airstrip on their property and I often used it for visits to nearby properties in the Kenepuru. One December afternoon I returned to the Pawnee to find a huge Christmas cake on the seat. No wonder I always came home from the Sounds with a warm feeling.

Food and friendship were not the only exports from the Sounds. Mary, the Bowrons' daughter, is also a vet and is now a valuable addition to the team at The Vet Centre in Blenheim. I like to think her choice of career was caused by something that might have rubbed off from my visits.

Other properties I frequently visited included those of Tony and Joy Redwood and Mike and Kristen Gerard, usually for routine-type work such as pregnancy testing cows, or in the case of the Gerards, visits have invariably been for the precious house cow struck with severe mastitis or calving difficulties. David and Rebecca Drake at Titirangi in the outer Sounds have a short, steep and quite challenging airstrip, especially in nor'westers, which a friend and I not infrequently fly to 'for the hell of it' and for a cup of tea in a unique and beautiful bay.

My calls to the Sounds properties were always memorable and I looked forward to them — less so if I had to drive which I found rather tedious. Occasionally we went by boat but if I could I always flew. That too wasn't without its mishaps. I have written about the problem I had landing at D'Urville Island in 'A Long Day on D'Urville' (page 73) and in *Cock and Bull Stories* you can read about the time the Piper Cub I flew into Clova Bay blew over and was written off while parked on the Gerards' airstrip. But I have enjoyed getting to know these wonderful characters and admired their tenacity for farming in a difficult but beautiful environment.

The Sounds also seems, when one appreciates the very small population living in the area, to have produced a disproportionate number of outstanding artists. No one can paint water like Rick Edmonds, nor portraits as can a very young self-taught extremely talented artist Rebekah Codlin. Award-winning authors from the Sounds include Joy Cowley, a prolific children's book writer, and Heather Heberley from the famous whaling family.

In recent times the Sounds seem to have attracted a wide range of characters from all over the globe. Perhaps it is the cheaper land, isolation, or a desire to get out of the rat race. I'm not sure but I do know I have experienced some interesting times with a number of them. Many of these folk would appear to have come from very busy and exciting lives in large cities and perhaps always dreamed of finding a quiet paradise by the sea. A lack of money does not seem to be an issue. On first meeting them I found they were invariably very excited about having shifted to this beautiful but remote part of the world and were not at all daunted by the isolation. In fact they seemed to have welcomed it as much as the friendly locals welcomed them. A few, however, turned out to be somewhat devious characters quietly trying to escape from a bad reputation acquired elsewhere in the country. The odd one arrived bringing some weird religion while others came because they found it an ideal climate to cultivate a certain herb.

Some bought lifestyle blocks while a few bought larger sheep and beef properties. One of the conditions for overseas buyers to purchase farms has been that the purchaser invested in the land and maintained the production coming off it. While a few have invested heavily in these properties and made them once again highly productive, this has not been honoured on one or two of the larger Sounds farms. These people have usually built huge mansions and perhaps improved the farm tracks but farming has been let go and much of the land has now, rightly or wrongly, started to revert to native bush. The property becomes their holiday retreat which they return to for a couple of weeks, once or twice a year.

Most of those taking up lifestyle blocks or smaller farms did so with the intention of making it their home. These were the ones with whom I had most of my dealings because, without exception, all seemed to 'love' animals, especially horses, but only a few had any real aptitude with them. Most did not seem to appreciate the difficulties isolation meant when it came to getting things done, particularly in an emergency. They were quite impressed and pleased with the fact that I could fly into the Sounds, often at short notice and in no time at all.

Unfortunately some were used to a system where things happen quickly and jobs get done to order and immediately, and they were incredibly intolerant and very demanding. One horse owner and new Sounds resident travelled for an hour and a half to a property where Rob Ander, one of our vets, was busy pregnancy testing a herd and forced him to leave the job immediately to attend to her horse with colic. Rob followed her home and determined the horse had a parasitic-induced colic. She insisted there was no way her animals had parasites and that her neighbour was trying to poison her horses and Rob was totally incompetent. She 'shooed' him off the place and Rob then had to drive an hour and a half back to finish the cows. We never tended to her horses again.

This woman never really appreciated the society she had shifted to, and was suspicious of outsiders or anyone showing an interest in her place or even going out of their way to be neighbourly. I could never understand why she thought anyone would want to poison her horses.

One couple who kept horses also had a stallion because they 'always wanted to breed horses'. For us, working with these animals could at times be a little difficult because they had never been handled properly and the colts never castrated. The breeding programme was soon out of control and I have no idea what they ever intended doing with the surplus animals. Selling unhandled horses is usually difficult and this couple cannot give them away because they 'love them too much'.

So there were some interesting times helping these newcomers from overseas and from New Zealand cities understand what was required to successfully keep horses and cows and sheep and deer. Many didn't have a clue and luckily for most of them, kind-hearted neighbours would always be there to give some guidance and a helping hand. Managing any animal is so much easier if the owner knows a little about animal behaviour and knows how to handle and work with them as farmers in general do. But dealing with those who move to the country with little or no previous experience with large animals adds another dimension to the job.

One couple had set up a reasonably large vineyard and farmed deer, both occupations that required hard-to-obtain help in the Sounds. Tiffany was a lovely young woman from Auckland who had spent recent years in California where she had been very involved in the wine industry. She brought her American husband back to New Zealand and bought a Sounds property that had around 200 deer running on it, including about 80 stags, as well as a few alpaca and a small flock of goats. She had also in a very short time of arrival acquired a Clydesdale gelding, a couple of hacks and several ponies varying in age and sex from young colts to an old wily arthritic mare. The delightful Tiffany obviously had this dream of owning a farm populated by a large menagerie, with the residents all happily living together and hadn't thought too much about the care and feeding of them. Someone mentioned that the horses and ponies needed their feet done and perhaps they should have their teeth checked as well and the colts should be castrated. So I arrived on the property not knowing what to expect but very quickly realised it was going to be a long afternoon. Tiffany had no idea what was involved but obviously thought the vet would and she wouldn't need to worry about how we caught them. The horses and ponies all inhabited the one largish paddock, there were no facilities like a decent set of stock yards, and few of them had been handled in recent times. As you can imagine it was a drawn-out job with two people, one of whom didn't really know how to help, catching these animals one by one and dealing with them.

I mentioned to her before flying back to Blenheim that she

would have to look at getting the velvet off the stags soon and to let me know when she had organised someone to help her get them in and sort out the ones that needed develveting. I would come out and remove the velvet over two or three visits. This time Tiffany was well organised. A poor neighbour had spent many hours getting all the stags crammed into the nicely cleaned-out deer shed but by the time I arrived a lot of the velvet was damaged. Luckily I had with me John Howie, a Scottish vet who was working for us. John had a wonderful sense of humour but at the end of that day he had lost it all. Because of the effort getting the stags in and the damaged velvet we decided to develvet all the deer that had velvet whether they were ready or not. Not an easy job with limited space and the logistical difficulties of releasing recovered stags and dealing with tranquilised ones. John was very much a cow man and had limited experience with deer and throughout the afternoon I could hear him mumbling about how much he hated working with deer. As far as I am aware he has never touched one since.

Others have attempted to farm sheep and beef organically — difficult in a higher humidity environment, kind to all types of parasite. Unfortunately too often farming organically has been a convenient excuse for not doing anything, with animal health suffering and animal welfare becoming an issue. This was the case with one professional couple from Wellington who, despite their obvious intelligence and high social status there, became an embarrassment to the locals. The health of their stock deteriorated through shocking management and neglect.

One woman had four horses that she housed in beautiful stables they had built and she fed and tended to them as if they were champion event horses. One was difficult to handle and another was very old and crippled with arthritis. She loved this horse so much that she had brought it with her from the States. I'm not sure if any of these horses were ridden or could even be ridden or that the owner could even ride. But she did love them and I always enjoyed rather amusing visits there. The facilities were magnificent and she and her husband treated me very well.

One evening I received a call from John the husband. He said that Genevieve was back in the States and that the local girl who was tending the horses had found the youngest, Ted, with what sounded over the phone like 'choke'. This is a condition where food, often hay, gets caught up in the oesophagus halfway to the stomach. While this is not usually fatal it is distressing for the horse. Sometimes it will spontaneously clear itself. However, John said that I had better come out because Genevieve would shoot him if anything happened to Ted. It was too late in the day to fly so to save the long drive he would come in by boat and pick me up in Havelock. This is what happened but by the time we got back to his place in the Kenepuru it was dark. The girl tending Ted was there to meet us and informed us that Ted was now OK and happily eating again. So we turned around and headed back to Havelock in his 9 metre twin outboard runabout at an incredible speed. It was so dark we couldn't see a thing but John navigated using his GPS unit, the first I had ever seen. It was probably one of the most nerve-wracking rides I have ever experienced in any mode of transport. I had horrible visions of hitting one of the large logs I had seen floating in the water on the way out. John did not seem at all concerned but I was very relieved when we got back to the 5 knot stretch of water nearer Havelock.

While these new Sounds residents have invariably added some colour to the area, and been fodder for a good laugh, many sadly have not lasted too long in the region. Some of their marriages have split up, and some have split up other marriages, and some in one way or another have eventually fallen out with a neighbour. Perhaps they have not understood the value of tolerance in long-term relationships. Essential if one wants to survive happily in remoter areas. Or perhaps they have just craved the social and easier life in the city. Some have returned to their homelands while others have shifted to New Zealand towns leaving their legacies — out of character mansions, a vineyard, and sometimes farms in poorer condition than when they took them over.

But really only a small percentage of newcomers to the farmed areas in the Sounds have not adapted. Most who have moved in during my time in practice have successfully farmed or semi-retired to smaller blocks while continuing to work in their professions, made possible by today's incredible means of communication. Some have made huge contributions improving the stock performance on the farms they have moved onto while others have improved the health of the land, ridding areas of wilding pines and encouraging the regeneration of native bush. These people, like those before them, appreciate the privilege and wonder of living in this beautiful and peaceful environment.

EMIL – PJ

I have to admit, here and now, that I have never been mad keen on dairy farming.

My early times on sheep farms in the South Island gave me a great love for the life, the country and the people. The freedom, the wide open spaces, the flexibility of times and places; things which all sheep and beef farmers and their workers will understand.

Then I spent five years at Lincoln College, now Lincoln University, getting a science degree in agriculture. That taught me a lot of things about land use and sustainable production systems. My education and all my subsequent experience taught me that land use options are based completely around what the soils and the water can cope with. Sheep and beef farming has always been based on those simple principles.

Dairy farming is very different. Regimented and scheduled, everything revolves around milking times, mostly twice a day. It's become a cornerstone of our economy now, even if the high-producing, high-cost structure (and high-debt model) is now looking a bit flawed, but it never appealed to me as a way of life. The people on those farms work their butts off, but not all of them see the big sustainable picture. If that turns some readers off now, I'm sorry. I don't apologise for discussing the principles I'm talking about.

My direct experience of working on a dairy farm took me, in 1969, to Tokoroa, heart of the timber industry, and also the heart of the Waikato dairy industry. I was 22 years old, fit and healthy. I'd already had a couple of years working on back-country sheep and beef farms, but as part of my first degree, a Bachelor of Agricultural Science, I had to do my time on a dairy farm.

Grant Turner, a friend from Lincoln College, found me the job on a farm next to his family's, just north of Tokoroa, and I arrived there in late November. It was a bit of a shock. The culture, the strict timetable dictated by milking times, the small scale in terms of acreage, all seemed foreign. (If I talk in acres rather than hectares, please excuse it as a sign of my age and education. I now embrace hectares, but in those days we all thought in acres.)

Dairy farming then was not what it is today. It was the dominant part of farming in the Waikato and Taranaki, but not in most of rural New Zealand. It was quite important economically but didn't match meat and wool on the big screen.

A sizeable herd was 200 cows, and the stocking rate might be one cow per acre, at best. Fertilisers were traditional with very little added nitrogen. Quite simply, it was more or less a sustainable model. There were certainly issues around direct contamination of streams, but no one took much notice. How the ground has changed.

I went to work for George Kuttel, a nice man of my own age,

a serious rally driver and a hay and silage contractor. George didn't spend much time on the farm; that was the lot of his younger brother Albert, a serious young man, shortly to be married; in fact he hitched up while I was there.

George and Albert lived in the family home with their father Emil and their mother, who I only ever knew as Mrs Kuttel. She was a fearsome creature, flinty eyed and sharp of tongue, and she ran the household with an iron rod. I have no doubt she was a good mother, but my admiration for her probably stops there.

Emil was a delight. In his sixties, he'd arrived in New Zealand as a young man from his native Switzerland, and his homeland was still important to him. He loved Swiss music, but he wasn't allowed to play it in the house. His solution lay in an old wind-up gramophone that he perched on the back seat of his 1950s black Humber Super Snipe. He would put the car in first gear about 11 each morning and crawl along the winding farm lane. It was lovely fertile volcanic ash country with rolling easy terrain, but with enough small hills to make it testing on a tractor. At various places on the track, where a tree gave some shade, he would park the great black beast. Then he'd triumphantly and carefully slip an old 78rpm record from its paper sheath and put it on the turntable. Very carefully he would put the gramophone arm with the old pointed needle on the outer edge of the now revolving record, hop into the front seat and listen blissfully to the songs of his homeland. He was in heaven, or nearly so, for a man needs a drink on a hot day. Emil loved a beer, but Mrs K wasn't going to allow the demon drink in her house.

Emil had a solution for that too. There was a series of drinking troughs at strategic places in the lane. In each of these Emil stashed a couple of bottles of DB brown ale, big bottles, with the long neck of the era. Nice and cool. With his Swiss music going and a glass of beer in hand, heaven was even closer. But not quite close enough. A dazzling ray of sunlight shone through the tree from time to time, spoiling his peace.

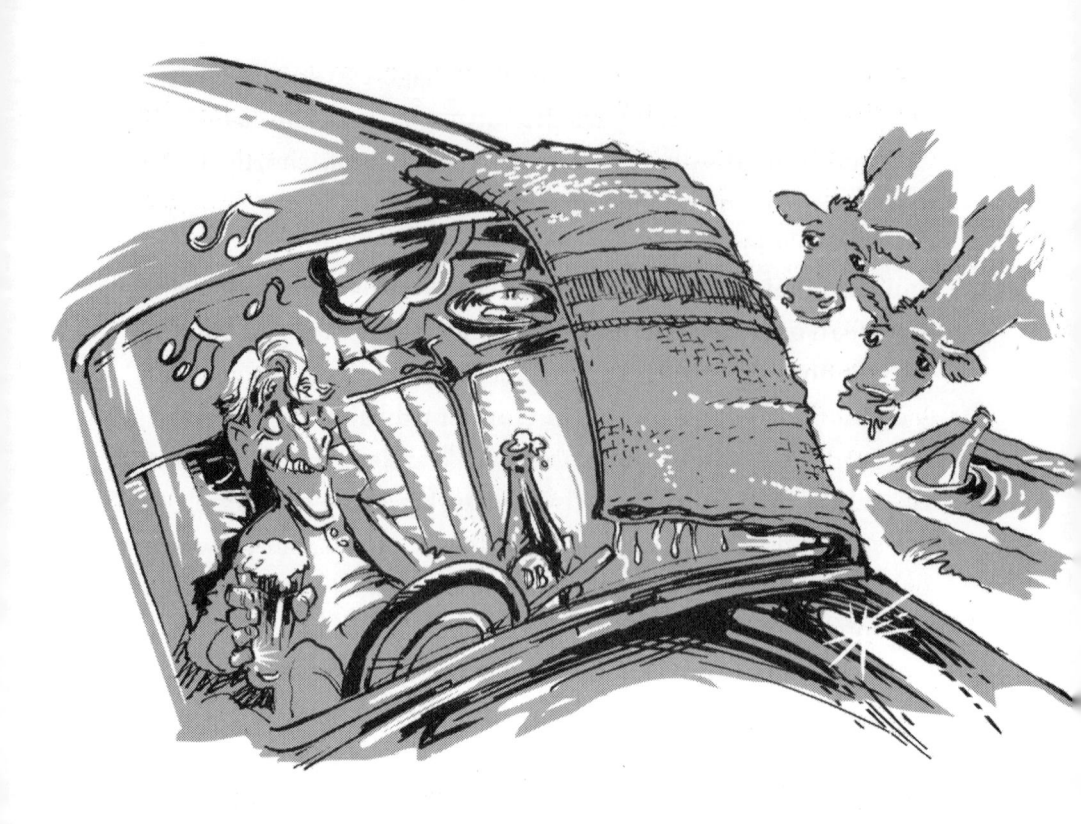

Solution three was an old wheat sack, a three striper, moistened in the trough then draped from the roof over the windscreen. Heaven was reached.

Many times in the three months I spent on that farm, I would see the old Snipe parked somewhere along the kilometre-long lane, sack on windscreen and music wafting from the open windows. The old boy would lie back and close his eyes, but his grip on the glass of beer never wavered.

For some reason, Emil took a shine to me. It may have been

because his wife didn't like me at all. Perhaps my face gave away the distaste for the boiled whole potato that sat on my plate for every meal, breakfast, lunch and dinner. The only variation was what went with it. Perhaps a piece of toast in the morning, a lettuce leaf at lunchtime, a chop at night.

Coming from South Island sheep and beef farms I was used to plenty of food, and I always felt hungry in Tokoroa. Whatever the reason, Mrs K didn't think much of me, but Emil became my friend.

On one occasion George decided I needed educating in the ways of Hamilton. We left the farm on a Saturday night and travelled at high speed up State Highway One through the little dairy town of Putaruru, and what we did in Hamilton I have no recollection of, but I remember a couple of bars. At 2 a.m. it was time to go home. I was milking and I had to get the cows in from four-thirty.

Somewhere around Cambridge, with rain on the windscreen, a wet road, and the speedometer showing around 150, George said, 'Watch this!' On a straight stretch of road he spun the wheel. The car did three, not one but three, 360 degree spins along the white line of the main highway, and when we'd stopped gasping, George the rally driver headed on home and delivered us to the farm.

Flick... 'Shit.'

Flick... 'Shit.'

Something was annoying the hell out of me. I'd lain down on the bed at 4 a.m., fully clothed, telling George I'd just have a rest before I went to get the cows. George, God bless him, had immediately climbed into the adjacent bed and gone to sleep. So, apparently, had I.

Flick... 'Bugger off.'

Flick … 'Fine man you have here, George.'

Flick.

'Fuck off,' or so George later told me that I'd mumbled.

Mrs Kuttel was standing by the bed, flicking water from a cup into my ear.

The boss lay in deep slumber less than a metre away, while his mother attacked the said fine employee, yours truly. It was 5.30 a.m. and milking was going to be late. I stumbled out, completely discombobulated, and somehow brought the cows in for milking but we probably missed the tanker.

Result: a 'grade'. Downgraded payout for the day. Shame on the hired hand.

After that I was dog tucker in Mrs K's eyes. The summer was a long one, relieved by the odd game of cricket (Sundays 9 a.m. to 3 p.m. in the Waikato), some evening hay-carting with locals, and the occasional foray with Emil.

One night, Mrs K went out, a rare occurrence. We all had our dinner, a sausage and a potato, then Mrs K packed her bag and disappeared. I don't think she could drive, so perhaps George took her or maybe a friend picked her up, because I was left alone in the house with Emil. He was a different man, cheerful and ebullient.

'Hey Pettterrr,' he said, 'would you like a trink?' His Swiss accent was thick and guttural, but warm and friendly. I thanked him, and he took me through to the living room, the holy of holies, where I'd never been invited before.

'Look,' he croaked. 'George brought me ziss from Ausstrallia.' With a flourish he pulled out a full bottle of Benedictine, a high-alcohol liqueur which many will recognise. 'Ve'd better haft one.'

He produced two huge glasses, the sort that peanut butter used to come in in the 1960s, about 300 millilitres in volume.

They were designed for household use as general drinking glasses once the peanut butter was gone.

He removed the screw top of the Benedictine bottle with difficulty, and filled the two glasses to the brim. I looked at the bottle as he put it down. It was two-thirds empty. 'Cheers,' he cried and, with a flourish, lifted his glass to his mouth and drained the lot, neat.

I watched, fascinated, as his eyes watered, his face went red, and his hands went to his head.

'Cheeesuss,' he cried, and disappeared out of the room. I could hear him crashing around in the bathroom, then he must have gone to his bedroom. I saw him no more. I carefully poured my glassful back into the bottle, and replaced the offending article in the cabinet.

I took the glasses to the kitchen, washed and dried them, and returned them to their cupboard. I looked around. No evidence for Mrs K. I closed the door and returned to my bedroom.

Never a word was said, but Emil wasn't at breakfast next day, and Mrs K seemed grimmer than ever. I felt a warm glow for this kind man. A good bugger.

But I would rather have been on a South Island sheep farm.

There is a postscript to this story. In early 2015 the phone rang at my home.

'Voice from the past,' said the unknown caller.

I had no idea who the voice belonged to. Which one of my old Lincoln mates was it? 'Give me a clue,' I ventured.

'You reckoned I couldn't drive a nail up a dead pig's arse,' from the mystery man.

Now that particular vulgar clause is one some Aussie taught

me years ago in Sydney, when I worked with some mechanics. I've often used it since as banter to many mates when they've made a minor driving error, or just to joke about their driving ability in general. The answer didn't help at all.

'Give me another clue, I'm stuck.'

'Greymouth,' he said. '1974.'

I still couldn't think who it was. I'd probably used the jibe a thousand times. It usually made people laugh.

'George Kuttel,' he said.

Bloody hell. George was Emil's son, the dairy farmer and hay and silage contractor and rally driver. I hadn't seen him for 45 years.

Now the Greymouth bit comes from when Ally and I were first married in 1972 and we went to live on the West Coast. I worked for the Westland Catchment Board as a soil conservator, and Ally taught at the local Catholic high school. The Rally of New Zealand came through the West Coast one weekend. I knew George was in it, so I went down to the Greymouth centre where all the cars were on display on Saturday. I found George's car, but I couldn't find George, so I'd left a note on his windscreen.

'Sorry to miss you, but you couldn't drive a nail etc, etc...'

I hadn't seen him since, but in 2015 George had been in a bookshop in Tauranga and seen *Cock and Bull Stories*. He'd recognised my name and bought it. Then he'd looked me up and rung me.

I was really chuffed. Forty-five years and we still had a bond.

Such is rural New Zealand.

BINKY BOYLE – PJ

Dogs. I've always loved them. As a child in Dunedin we had a bad-tempered family cocker spaniel called Jamie, who bit so many people he was eventually put down, but he didn't put me off dogs.

When I went to work on farms it was a joy to have my very own dogs, to train and spend most of my working day with them.

As a veterinarian I found I had a natural affinity with dogs, and I got on pretty well with most of them. And yet, looking back, without being reminded, I can only remember a few as individuals. Apart from those we owned as a family of course.

Of the individuals I do remember, one standout was Binky Boyle. Really there was nothing particularly standout about him, but there was something very special about his owners.

Binky himself came to us in 1998, not long after we opened the new clinic in Redwood Street with Stuart Burrough. I think he may have been Stuart's patient at his previous practice, but I'm not really sure. Over the next nine years we all saw Binky regularly. He was a solid little bichon frise, who had many of the standard mishaps in his life.

A ruptured right anterior cruciate ligament. A corneal ulcer. Then a ruptured left anterior cruciate a year later, a not uncommon problem for dogs. Persistent ear infections. Skin infections on his abdomen which turned out to be food allergy, and so on. In later life Binky prolapsed a lumbar disc, developed moderate hypothyroidism, and was put on ACE inhibitors to treat his elevated blood pressure.

None of these things are unusual in a dog's life. But his owners were simply extraordinary.

Raewyn and Don Boyle were and are good ordinary New Zealanders. There was nothing flash about them, and I'm sure they live straightforward and decent, simple lives, still.

They would do anything for Binky, and brought him to the clinic regularly. In later years they would have up to 20 visits to the clinic in a year, and we had a solid, friendly relationship with them both.

What made them very special was chocolate. Raewyn Boyle made chocolates to a standard as high as most whose whole business is chocolates.

She made thousands of them, in myriad shapes. She must have had hundreds of moulds, and her skills were wondrous.

Raewyn didn't sell any of her chocolates, she gave them away. And The Vet Centre Marlborough was one of the greatest beneficiaries of her generosity. Three or four times a year Raewyn would appear in the clinic with a massive basket of chocolates, sometimes two.

Their presentation was superb. Coloured ribbons and tinsel,

Father Christmases, reindeer, Easter bunnies, you name it, Raewyn made it. There were solid chocolates, chewy chocolates and chocolates with a huge variety of delicious soft fillings. Every basket was labelled 'From Binky Boyle'.

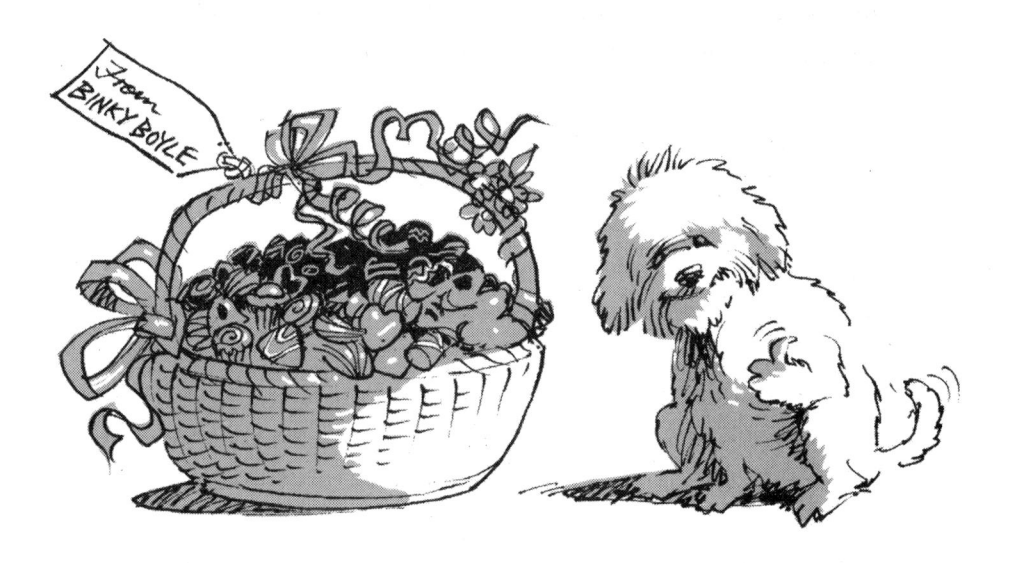

There would be whoops of delight in the staffroom as the receptionist arrived holding the latest wonder from Binky, and so large were the offerings that it usually took several days for a dozen hungry nurses and vets to clean them all up.

Raewyn's generosity was amazing, and her skill in making the chocolates was extraordinary. I never found out whether Raewyn and Don had grandchildren, but if they did they must have thought gallons of chocolate was normal life.

From time to time Binky would turn up for another appointment, never very happy about being there, but stoically enduring whatever latest indignity we were putting him through, whether it was a thermometer up his bottom, some fluorescein in his eye, or blood being taken from his cephalic vein in the front leg. He never grumbled, but neither did he look excited to see us.

There has never been another Raewyn Boyle and probably never will be. She and Don loved Binky passionately, and the chocolates were their way of showing they appreciated our care.

It's generosity like theirs which puts the icing on the cake for us veterinarians. We did our jobs as professionally as we could, and the successful outcome of whatever we were doing was reward in itself. But the amazing and special relationships we formed with people made worthwhile all the long hours, the late calls and the working weekends.

Just before I retired in 2007, Don and Raewyn made an appointment for Binky, and they wanted me to see him. At that stage Binky was developing mild Cushings disease. This is a chronic over production of corticosteroids from the adrenal gland, and is life threatening. He was in his twelfth year, and was drinking and urinating a lot, and the Boyles were worried for him. He was getting pretty lethargic and I knew he didn't have long to go. But he was still interested in life around him, and it wasn't yet his time.

As the consultation finished, Don Boyle said, 'You might like this, Pete. It's our thank you.' From a bag he produced a wrapped bottle. I unwrapped it there and then. It was a litre of Wilson's whisky, New Zealand made. Somehow they had known of my liking for the malt.

It was another example of their amazing kindness, and I

struggled with the lump in my throat as I thanked them and said my goodbye.

I'm struggling with it again as I write this story.

It was wonderful people like Don and Raewyn who have left me with lasting memories of a life as a vet.

THE TELEPHONE CALL — PA

Invariably contact with clients, whether to arrange a visit or to discuss some issue, is via the telephone. Knowing who it is you are actually about to talk to has some real advantages. I was always very grateful if the receptionist at work or a family member at home had found out the name of the person who wanted to speak to me. It did influence the way I answered the phone. However, it wasn't always that simple.

One receptionist at work was never really cut out to be a telephonist. She either never found out who it was or, when she did, by the time she had directed the call to me she had forgotten who it was or got the name wrong. Others were very good and sometimes would even apologise that I was unavailable when they knew I wasn't in the right frame of mind to talk to that particular client.

My wife Diana, who no one knows as Diana because since she was a very young child her father started calling her Chick (because she spent all day watching the chooks at the bottom of their garden), was great on the phone and always answered it stating her name. However, nothing infuriated her more than the clients — and there were two in particular — whose first words after she answered the phone were 'Peter there?' No 'Hello Chick, it's John X here. Wonder if I could speak to Peter please.' While she got to know exactly who they were as soon as they said 'Peter there?' she always made a point of asking for their name. They never got the hint, and as a result I would invariably get the phone thrust at me by a teeth-gritting fuming spouse. If only people understood that if they wanted a good response from someone they were after for advice or help, then how they introduced themselves had a huge effect on the response they got — at least from me.

On several occasions I have been guilty of not knowing who I was talking to despite them introducing themselves. It was easy enough if I didn't know the person — I just knew I was talking to someone I didn't know. But when I should have known who it was and couldn't place them it could get awkward. The longer you delayed getting around to admitting you didn't quite get their name or didn't know who it was you were talking to, the harder it got. I have on occasions got through a whole conversation trying to fit the name to a face and place, and yet was confident the person I was talking to was oblivious of my predicament.

One Saturday morning Chick called me into the house and handed me the phone.

'Rob Todd needs to talk to you.' A quizzical look on her face as if she and I should both know who Rob Todd was.

'Good morning.'

'Good morning, Pete, how are you — Rob Todd here.'

'Good morning, Rob.'

Who the hell is Rob Todd? Bob Todd? No, I don't know a Bob

Todd nor a Robert Todd. Could it be Bob Todhunter? No it's not him — I know him well and it definitely doesn't sound like him. 'How can I help, Rob?'

'It's bloody footrot, Pete. Every year my merino hoggets get footrot and I can never clear it up.'

Ah — so Rob Todd is a merino farmer. He is not a Marlborough merino farmer because I know them all well, so he must be one from down south and someone I have bumped into on one of my trips to Otago. I have a handful of good merino farmer clients in the Omarama–Wanaka area and perhaps he was a neighbour of one of them. He had a ring of authority in his voice and I immediately got the impression he had probably been farming in the high country all his life. His voice also suggested that he was not a young farmer, but one who had probably lived with footrot in his flock most of his farming career and had finally come to the realisation that what he was doing and had always done to get on top of the disease was perhaps not the right approach. Maybe word had spread that I had had some involvement with footrot and some success in helping farmers understand and control the disease.

Footrot is the bane of merino farmers' lives. Unless treated it will cause severe and painful lesions in a sheep's foot and cripple them. It is a highly infectious bacterial disease and spreads under warm damp conditions. The merino and other fine-wool breeds derived from the merino are genetically more susceptible to footrot than others, and mainly for this reason their distribution is limited to the drier areas of the country. Unless a well set-up programme to identify infected sheep, or more importantly to identify non-infected sheep and keep them isolated, is adhered to then the disease will remain in the flock for years. Too often farmers spend far too long in paring and treating infected sheep in inadequate facilities, employing uncommitted staff who hate the job because they know they will be doing the same back-breaking thankless task the same time again next year. Footrot really is a horrible disease with serious impacts on flock performance, and for this reason extensive research is currently under way to identify resistant animals and their genetic markers. It is obviously extremely painful for the animal and quite possibly, if left untreated, a far more important welfare issue than some of the conditions we inflict on sheep such as tailing (tail docking) or even shearing that certain animal rights groups in their ignorance go on about.

Meanwhile, my approach with farmers is to help them organise a control programme. Invariably before a good programme can be initiated a good facility has to be built. This will involve a bath to wash the feet before inspecting them, a sheep handler to tip the sheep up so that the feet can be inspected properly, and a shallow soak bath where groups of sheep can be stood in a solution, usually of zinc sulphate, to bathe and treat the feet.

By now I suspected that Rob was a Canterbury or Otago high country merino farmer, perhaps 5000-6000 ewes and possibly a wether flock as well, and running 2000-3000 hoggets. Because those who have trouble controlling the disease have almost always got poorly designed and built handling set-ups, if any at all, he is bound to have inadequate facilities.

'So what sort of facilities have you got and how have you been treating them, Rob?'

'I really haven't got too much in the way of facilities.' I was right. 'I just catch them when they limp and squirt footrot stuff I got from the vet clinic on their feet. Doesn't seem to help much though.'

Bloody hell. How does he expect to get on top of the problem if that is all he is doing? He will only be treating a fraction of the mob if all he is doing is treating the 'limpers' — the ones with the most severe footrot. Most of the flock might only have a mild foot infection and not be limping noticeably at all, or have it in more than one foot. It is very hard to limp when both feet hurt!

'So every year your hoggets get footrot badly. How are they now?'

'I've got rid of them all now. None left. All gone to the works.'

Rob was obviously a desperate man. Solved the problem by quitting all his replacements. Probably not a bad idea under the circumstances, but nevertheless it was still a drastic measure to sell all his replacements. I needed to arrange a visit soon and spend some time talking about the disease and how to set up a robust footrot control programme. There was an opportunity here!

'So how many hoggets do you normally run and what about the ewes?'

'Usually about 1800 and I don't run any ewes.'

Things are falling into place. I'm beginning to build up a profile of Rob but still can't place him. Rob has to be running a large wether flock and every year he buys in 1800 replacement wether lambs. With that number coming in, and after selecting out the best ones to go into the flock, he is probably running a large wether flock of 7000-8000 animals. Some of the harder high country farms run smallish ewe flocks simply to breed lambs to replace those wethers which die from natural causes or are culled for age or for other reasons. The only source of income from these flocks is their valuable fine merino wool. Some like Rob just buy in replacements and don't have a ewe flock. But where the hell is he? He has to be the owner or manager of one of the larger, harder, more remote high country properties, somewhere in the Otago or Canterbury back country. These large runholders are invariably proud independent sorts who rarely call on advice from vets. Partly I suspect because they think it is a sign of weakness and partly because some of them do not believe we understand their business. Anyway I really needed to get a clue about who this desperate man was.

'Rob — this might require more than a phone call to get on top of. I wonder if it wouldn't be best if I sat down with you and set up a control programme. Can you remind me how best to get to your property? I assume you have an airstrip on the place.'

There was a moment's silence on the end of the phone. 'Appleby. Pete, you should remember, you've been here enough.'

Appleby!

Appleby is a district a few kilometres south of Nelson. There are no merino flocks in Appleby. It is an area of fertile soils with small lifestyle blocks, orchards, vineyards and market gardens. Rob Todd from Appleby in market garden country. Then it came to me.

'Toddy!'

Toddy and Trish are a wonderful couple and are very good friends of Chick's sister and brother-in-law Ju and Philip, and they run a market garden in Appleby. We had got to know them over the years but he was always just Toddy. Never knew him as Rob Todd. It so happened that every year Toddy would buy in around 18 merino lambs and use them to clean up grass and weeds around his market garden. He preferred merinos over other breeds because they were more respectful of his substandard fences and didn't eat all the vegetables.

'Toddy — you could have told me it was you. Here I am thinking I am talking to this important Otago high country merino farmer Robert Todd, potentially a valuable new client and it's you — a bloody market gardener from Appleby running 18 miserable footrotty merinos.'

We had a good chuckle and I know my sister-in-law dined out on the story for months.

Nowadays Toddy is known as the Appleby merino farmer.

BEASTLY – PJ

In the mid-1980s when Rogernomics had let the grey shoe brigade loose in the financial markets, one of the benefits for us vets was the money that business people, mostly city-based, were prepared to punt. And one of the entrepreneurial schemes which attracted these people was embryo transfer in goats, sheep and deer. As we've mentioned elsewhere in 'Angora Anguish' (page 47) and 'Helping the Ram Out' (page 169), Pete A and I got ourselves educated in this highly technical business, and became firmly involved.

This meant that for a couple of months in April and May we were busier than we could cope with. For the rest of the year the business was the right size for two of us, and being Marlborough, and mostly dry land conservative farming, the situation didn't justify us getting another full-time vet just then. The answer lay in veterinary locums. For the three or four years of the goat boom we would hire a locum vet to look after the practice while we were out doing embryo transfer (ET).

Some were very good, others were not. One of the early locums had a habit of making the nurses take the X-rays while he left the building, so he wouldn't be exposed to the radiation. We only found that out after he'd gone. He wasn't employed again.

The very best one we got was a delightful Englishman named Pete Orpin. The only downside was that it meant there were three Petes in the practice, and it could get a bit confusing. Pete O came to us through an agency. His CV said he played rugby, so he was more than halfway in the door. It also said he could juggle and eat an apple at the same time. That sealed it. We employed him without an interview.

He turned out to be as good as he promised. He and his lovely Glaswegian wife Bronwen arrived in Blenheim and rented a flat for three months. He was a good small animal vet and a very good large animal one. And he could indeed juggle as he'd claimed. Especially when he'd had a few beers.

Bronwen worked as my technician when I did laparoscopic artificial insemination in sheep, another practice I was heavily involved in. (She was the one who'd say 'Blow, don't suck' to herself as she emptied the straws.) She was also a good musician, and quickly became part of the folk music community in the region. She was a funny, delightful person to be around.

Bronwen and Pete O had only been married a few months, and their bright outward-looking attitude and friendly personalities saw them become our firm friends. Thirty years later we still keep in touch, and have visited each other many times. They live near Leicester in the Midlands where Pete is principal of a large practice, and they've raised four smart and interesting children.

Pete O's one missing area of expertise was in deer. There was no commercial deer farming in the UK then, and New Zealand was very much leading the world. Pete A and I had been in it from the start, and had many deer farm clients. We were reasonably confident deer vets when Pete Orpin arrived. TB testing of deer herds was a significant part of our work in those days, and Pete O was keen to learn. The industry had been established mostly from captured wild deer, and TB was a real problem in some of those. It was a very fast-growing industry, and deer were bought and sold, often rapidly, and sent all over the country. The result was that TB spread rapidly, and became a national problem.

TB testing involved shaving some fur from the side of the animal's neck to get a patch of bare skin, and injecting a tiny dose of Tuberculin into the skin. Three days later we had to return to the farm and view and palpate the area to see if there was a reaction to the Tuberculin. If there was, it could mean the animal was infected. If so, it had to be slaughtered and post-mortemed. It was a necessary but unpopular management practice. It was also hard work, and worse, the reliability of the test was not 100 per cent. Healthy animals could give a positive result, and end up being slaughtered unnecessarily. For vets it was either a good or bad job depending on the shed facilities and, consequently, how easy it was to handle the deer, to clip them, inject and read them. Deer are very sensitive animals, and the noise of the electric clippers could be very frightening for them. In good, well set-up sheds, it was a pleasant job. But not every farmer had such sheds.

On one day in May or June, we sent Pete Orpin off to TB test a herd of deer belonging to the Bristed brothers, aka the Fuzzy Brothers. Bill and Dick Bristed are legendary Marlborough characters. Identical twins, they've fooled a lot of traffic cops, and a lot of other people too. The normal rules of engagement, particularly bureaucratic ones, are not something the brothers subscribe to, and their TB testing scene was not of the highest standard. The deer shed at Cobden Farm near Seddon was made from old packing cases, hastily banged together at minimal cost. The gates, a vital part of a deer shed with these highly strung and powerful animals, were old house doors, the hinges nailed to the door frames (what door frames?) with bent-over three inch nails, one or two per hinge.

What's more, the Bristeds didn't just have red deer. They had a herd of fallow deer, small but explosive, and almost impossible to handle. Worse still, they had wapiti, the very large cousin of the red deer. A wapiti bull or cow in confined quarters is a very dangerous opponent and their swinging front legs, or their immensely powerful back ones, can inflict a lot of damage on a human, especially a veterinary one.

The Bristeds' herds were known to the Ministry of Agriculture vet as having a few TB problems, not least because the numbers never added up, or equated to previous tests. In short it was a bureaucrat's nightmare, and only just better for the rest of us. The upside was the Bristeds are good buggers, and I always enjoyed the entertainment when I went there, once I knew and understood how they worked.

So we sent Pete Orpin to do the TB testing, big strong lad that he was, and he went off in high spirits, ready to tackle a new job. At 6 p.m. Pete and I were in the clinic, cleaning up from whatever we'd been doing. I'd probably been doing small animals, and Pete might have been pregnancy testing cows, but it could well have been the other way round.

What I do remember is a very ragged, bruised and dirty Pete Orpin bursting into the clinic, eyes glazed, hair awry. He looked shocked. 'Don't ever send me to those bloody Beastly Brothers again. It was a nightmare,' he muttered. He'd been bashed to bits by stroppy deer in the less-than-adequate shed, and he had had enough. We gave him a beer and sat him down, and in an hour he was back to normal.

We never sent him to work with the Bristeds again. But we often laughed at his name for them — the Beastly Brothers.

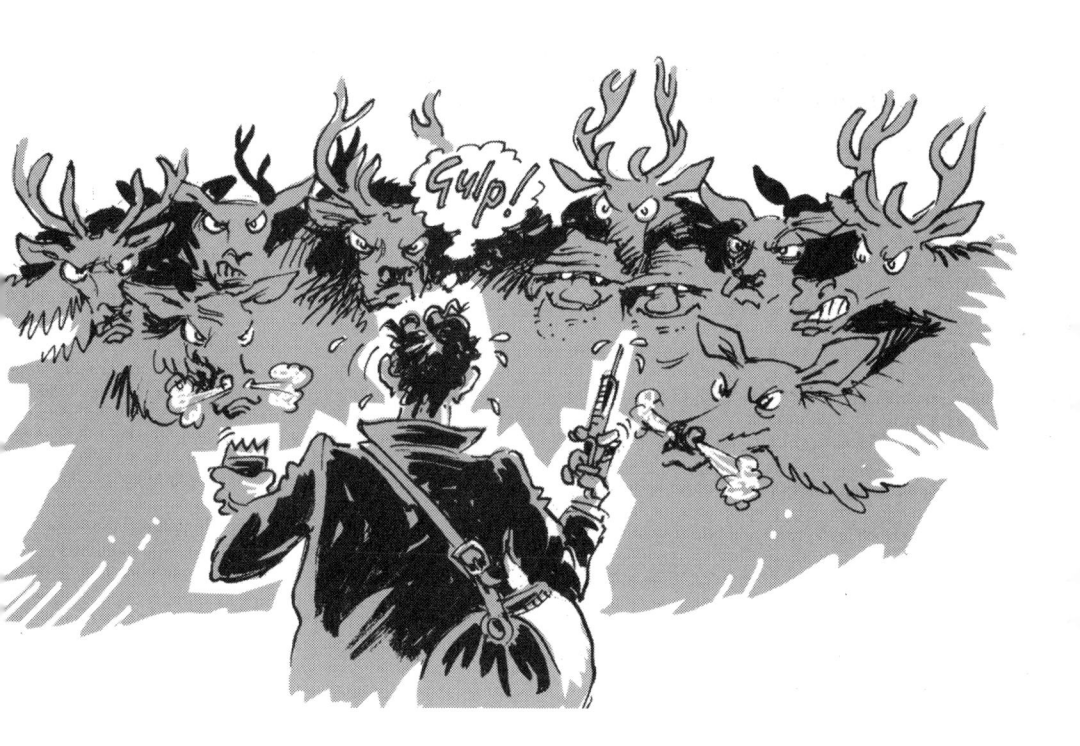

TRUSTING RELATIONSHIPS — PA

Trust, faith and confidence all describe the high regard one person has for another. These qualities are essential for veterinarians to maintain a good stable working relationship with our clients. Trust means a client believes in their vet's work and that he or she will do the right thing. Faith is more to do with the inner qualities of the vet — that he or she is a good person and that the client likes him or her. Both these qualities can be established fairly quickly, perhaps after a visit or two. Confidence, on the other hand, which depends more on a person's repeated experiences with the vet, can take a long time to establish.

So while the confidence that a pet owner or farmer has in their vet might have taken many years to develop, a single incident can wreck this wonderful relationship instantly. Sometimes the incident is the result of an unfortunate mistake or a bad decision by the vet, while at other times it may just be bad luck. Or a loss of confidence can be brought about by a different interpretation of an event or poor understanding by the client of the complexity of some of the issues we deal with. Too often, however, a poor outcome is simply the result of bad communication and perhaps a lack of empathy shown by the vet.

During 40 years of being a veterinary practitioner I have lost the odd client. It happens to us all. Sometimes I have no idea why. You just don't see that client any more and you hear that he or she now uses another vet. It could have been due to a loss of trust or confidence in my abilities or it could have been simply because that person just liked another vet more.

In my early days in practice there were far greater opportunities for things to go wrong. Not only was I inexperienced but I was also having a go at doing everything in all species. As vets, every one of us can probably think back to an incident that makes us inwardly shudder, that we wished we had managed better, and that lost us a client.

One of the great advantages of working in a smaller rural area is that after you have been there a while you know most of your clients, and when they ring you for advice or help they do so with confidence that you will do the right thing, otherwise they would ring another vet. They are prepared to listen and accept what you tell them. On the other hand people who don't know you ring anticipating a good outcome, hoping that you will immediately respond the way they expect you to. Sometimes when you don't react the way they are hoping you will they are disappointed. Occasionally you can lose a potential client before you have even met them.

One evening around 8 p.m., while on after hours duty and just settling down to my evening meal with Chick and our two children, I received a phone call.

'Hello. Peter Anderson speaking.'

'My pet rat needs to be put to sleep.' It's a boy and he is straight into it. No mucking around with any formalities.

'Oh dear. And what is wrong with your rat?'

'He's old and he's got a big growth on his face.'

Clearly neither of these things had developed between the clinic closing at 6 p.m. and now. It is hardly an emergency and the rat can wait until tomorrow. 'OK. That's no good. Would you like to bring him in tomorrow morning?'

After no immediate reply but some muffled voices in the background I again asked, 'Will tomorrow morning suit you?'

Another pause and then, 'I want to have him put to sleep now.'

He was obviously conferring with a higher power.

'Well, I could see your rat soon and do the job but I'm afraid that will cost you $50 if you want me to look at him tonight.'

Again there is no immediate reply and then a furious-sounding woman comes on the phone. 'What do you mean you won't look at my boy's pet tonight? I'm disgusted with your attitude.'

Naturally I was a little taken aback by this response but replied as calmly as I could. 'I'm sorry but I didn't say I wouldn't see him. I told your boy I could but it would cost him $50. I am not spending the next hour driving over 20 kilometres and opening up the clinic and putting his old rat to sleep with a condition that isn't an emergency and that could wait another 12 hours — for nothing.'

I thought that was reasonable but she was getting really angry now and was on a roll. 'What sort of vet are you? The last time we had to have a rat put to sleep the vet did it straight away and it didn't cost anything. I'm disgusted. You are a disgrace to the vetinry profession. I'm going to report you to the vetinry council.'

After that outburst I was momentarily stuck for words, but that didn't matter because the phone went dead in my ear. I went and sat down for my dinner somewhat bemused. I didn't really enjoy my meal after that.

We never did see the rat and I never did hear from the vet council. I have heard that rats make great pets but for some reason I have never been a great fan of this idea. Nevertheless my response would have been the same if the pet had been a cat or dog — I think!

The rat's owner's mother lost faith in me being a nice kind person before I had even met her. I certainly hadn't lived up to her expectation that I would solve their problem by immediately coming and putting her boy's poor old rat out of his misery — for nothing. I suspect it never occurred to her that I, too, like to sit down at the end of the day and have a pleasant dinner with my family, rather than driving to the clinic and opening it up for a non-emergency.

I remember a night in my early days of practice when I convinced Chick that we should go and watch a good movie that was on at the theatre. She is not a great fan of movies, unless they are exceptional, because when the lights go out she tends to fall asleep . . . I was always keen on Westerns in my younger days and naturally thought everyone else was too, including Chick. During our courtship, to give her a great night out, I would invest my meagre student allowance in a couple of tickets to the movies and get thoroughly engrossed in the cowboys and Indians, totally oblivious to the fact that Chick had fallen asleep among all the gunfire.

So it was an achievement to get her to this film. Just before the lights went out an elderly couple I knew moved along the row and sat down immediately in front of us. I remembered them well because I had treated Steph, a little bichon frise of theirs, a couple of weeks earlier. They were very worried because their little dog had been 'off-colour' for a day or so and I remembered it showed some abdominal pain and had a slight temperature and some diarrhoea, but really did not appear to be too ill. The dog responded well to an intravenous anti-inflammatory, becoming more relaxed and appearing happy enough. Despite the owners' continuing concern I sent them home with some antibiotics for Steph, reassuring them that it was just a mild upset tummy and she had probably eaten something that didn't agree with her. I also remember they weren't that happy when they left, mumbling something about it being nonsense that she would have eaten something she shouldn't have.

Anyway, come half-time at the movies, something they don't seem to have these days, I leaned forward and said to the couple over their shoulders, 'Hi, how are you? Great film isn't it? How's Steph doing?'

They obviously knew who they had sat in front of. She didn't respond but kept looking ahead at the commercials on the screen. He turned around slowly and said to me with obvious bitterness, 'She died, didn't you know?'

It had been a good film up until then. I had obviously made a poor decision about Steph, who must have had more than a mild enteritis. Certainly her owners had lost any confidence they had in me but I don't think they ever trusted me right at the beginning.

Bruce Taylor, my former classmate, a very well respected horse vet and an expert in equine reproduction with extensive experience in the USA, tells a story about a falling out of favour with one of his best clients.

Bruce, a partner in a large mixed practice in Rangiora, was

asked by Mr and Mrs Baxter to euthanase their old, very obese male donkey at Ohoka, a nearby district. Their children had all grown up with this donkey Eeyore and he was very much part of the family. The Baxters were very good clients. Bruce had done most of their veterinary work for years and he had an excellent relationship with them. He was definitely their 'favourite' vet. It was arranged that the unpleasant task would be done by Bruce on his own at 8 a.m. on a Monday, the Baxters choosing to be well away from home while this was performed. They had also arranged for a digger to come at nine, after Eeyore had been 'put to sleep' so he could be put in his final resting place.

After administration of the usual drug, a high concentration of the anaesthetic pentobarbitone, Eeyore duly dropped to the ground and stopped breathing. Bruce then travelled on to his next job, about 35 kilometres away, which would take up most of the rest of the morning. A couple of hours after arriving there he received a call from the clinic and couldn't believe what he was hearing.

He was informed that Mrs Baxter had returned home only to find Eeyore looking over the fence at her as she came up the drive — very much not dead. The digger had already come and gone without being able to find any body lying around anywhere to bury, so hadn't dug any hole. To say the Baxters were not best pleased is an understatement. Bruce's partner was asked to go out and do a 'proper' job and Bruce was definitely no longer the favourite vet. He never returned to the Baxters. I guess, perhaps understandably, they lost confidence in him! Bruce was not allowed to forget the incident with the indestructible Eeyore and had to shout beer all round for the partners and staff at the clinic.

Mark Wiseman, the bloke who set fire to a historic barn,

went on another farm visit on that same island to see his first sick sheep. She hadn't moved or eaten for 24 hours. Fresh from vet school, Mark was keen to perform a thorough clinical examination, which he duly did. Apart from the fact that she seemed unable to stand and uninterested in eating he could find nothing wrong with her. She didn't have a fever, no signs of respiratory disease, no obvious pain, no broken legs or sore hooves, she wasn't carrying or nursing lambs, nor were there any discharges from any orifices. The farmer didn't seem keen to spend money on blood tests so Mark had to pronounce that he could find nothing that needed treatment, but if she couldn't stand or eat the best thing to do was to put her to sleep. The farmer seemed happy with this advice as it cost him no extra money. Mark left with the plan that the farmer would shoot the sheep.

Some weeks later Mark bumped into this farmer who asked him if he remembered the sick sheep he had condemned to death. He told Mark he hadn't had a chance to do the deed until late that afternoon. However, as he approached the sheep she took one look at him with the gun and promptly jumped to her feet, ran off and had never looked back since!

Mark reckons this was his first lesson that we don't know all the answers and to never underestimate nature. Sometimes nature just needs a little time to sort itself out, and that thought has stayed with him throughout his career.

I can certainly relate to what happened to Mark; I may have approached it differently but nevertheless not handled it any better. Too often we feel that we are not doing our job or are not seen to being doing a good job unless we give the patient something. Early in my career, when faced with cases like Mark's, I would on occasions find myself thinking, 'Buggered if I know what is going on here. What the hell can I give this animal?'

Trusting Relationships | 235

I would usually resort to a shot of multivitamins or general tonic because these would at least be unlikely to cause any harm and they might help. While the farmer with the miraculously recovered sheep may not have been entirely confident in Mark's abilities he would have been able to dine out at Mark's expense for many months and I am sure would have been happy to have him back on the property again. On the other hand, if Mark had given the ewe a shot of vitamins, the farmer would have had a very different opinion of Mark's competence, despite the fact that the vitamins probably had little influence on her recovery.

So a 'tincture of time' can be the best treatment in many situations and we shouldn't be afraid of prescribing it. While vets often feel it is expected that we prescribe something or give some advice, doing nothing should not mean a client loses confidence in our abilities to do the right thing. But it is important we spend the time ensuring clients understand our course of action. Too often it is just easier and quicker to give an animal a jab of 'this' or suggest the flock get a drench with 'that', with little explanation required.

Communicating our course of action, whatever it might be, is so crucial. Regardless of the outcome it will often mean the difference between a client gaining or losing confidence and trust in us. In the end poor communication with the client is the main reason why there are breakdowns in good vet–client relationships.

NORWEGIANS WOULD — PJ

In 2003 I went on a sabbatical. It was something the principals had decided on early in the new practice that we formed in 1998 with Stuart Burrough. I can't recall the frequency, but the agreement was that each of the three principals, Pete A, Stuart and myself, would from time to time be awarded a three-month break from the practice, on full pay. An overseas trip in search of veterinary knowledge or skills which could be brought back to the practice was part of the deal, but it was meant to refresh and rekindle enthusiasm for the job.

When it came to my turn in 2003, I was already heavily involved in extending my knowledge and practice in dog reproduction. One of the top people in the world in that field was Professor Catharina Linde-Forsberg at the university in Uppsala, Sweden. I had already met Catharina at a three-day dog insemination workshop in 2000, also in Uppsala. She had offered me the chance to do further research, so I decided that that would be the basis for my sabbatical.

An added attraction was that our daughter Jane was studying advanced engineering geotechnics in Grenoble, France. And, to top it off, my good friend Neil Reid agreed to come to Scotland with me for a fortnight, studying malt whisky distilleries and golf courses. So it was lining up to be a pretty good trip.

Sweden had a further attraction for me. On my first visit I had met a delightful local who had spent some years in New Zealand. Claes Cedeström is a charming and gregarious companion, hugely travelled, well read and a keen sportsman. On the first occasion I had met him at a golf course beside Stockholm Airport when the AI course in Uppsala had finished. We played nine holes, then went for lunch in the clubhouse.

'Will you have a beer?' he enquired. I would, and in no time a pint, frosted and clear, was at the table. Then his arrived, a half pint. I didn't say much, but I played very badly in the second nine, and Claes won the match easily.

A year later when Claes visited New Zealand I commented on that game and the fact he only had a half pint to my pint. 'Oh yes,' said Claes, 'and yours was 7.5 per cent. Mine was light beer, 2 per cent.' Thanks Claes.

Back on the sabbatical I spent a pleasant week at the university with Catharina and her colleagues. I have to say that there wasn't a lot going on in the dog AI field that week, so I spent a bit of time in Uppsala, watching people go by. I came to realise that up to a certain point in a young person's life their face is bright and open, the corners of the mouth turned up.

Then somewhere in the mid- to late twenties there's a change. It may be to do with jobs, responsibilities, or having children, but there is a definite change to a more closed face, eyes less open, mouth turned down at the corners. It gave me food for thought.

When the week was up, I travelled on the train back to Stockholm and transferred to the Tullinge line where I was met at the station by Claes and his 17-year-old daughter Sophie, and off we went for a few days on their farm, south of Stockholm.

Then we took off across Sweden on a golfing trip. We played at some fantastic courses as we travelled west over several days, staying in hotels and backpackers. We moved into the mountains near the border with Norway, where we met Lapps, that nomadic group of people who own and herd reindeer, and after a week we passed over into Lillehammer. From there we drove high over the Norwegian mountains, bare and forbidding, reminiscent of our own Fiordland, and came down to the wonderful Sandefjord. It's magnificent scenery, and the population is low. I felt very much at home.

Finally we drove back to Oslo through a tunnel 27 kilometres long, an experience in itself, and arrived at the house of Claes' cousin Janna. She was a nice woman in her late forties, her husband a bearded Viking. We stayed the night in their home, with their four children from teenage down.

Klaus, the husband, was welcoming in a challenging sort of way. 'From New Zealand, eh?' he said. There was something about the way he said it that made me feel a bit less than welcome.

Klaus prepared trout, a small fish for each of us, beautifully cooked and presented. He poured each of us a drink, schnapps, small and powerful. We ate and sipped, the children very much part of the conversation. Their Uncle Claes was here, and his friend from far off New Zealand, and it was an occasion.

Then Klaus finished his schnapps. He reached for the bottle and poured himself another. My glass was finished too, and also Claes', but Klaus either didn't notice, or didn't care. He finished that one quickly, then another, and a fourth.

The conversation around the table was humming. The children wanted to know about New Zealand, and Janna and Claes had a lot of family things to catch up on.

Klaus, meanwhile, had lapsed into silence. Clearly drinking schnapps was not something one could do at the same time as talking. He finished his sixth glass and suddenly spoke.

'So, New Zealanders don't like us killing whales, eh?' He looked intensely at me, his eyes already bloodshot.

'Oh, I'm not sure we should go there tonight,' I responded. I certainly didn't want an argument as a guest in someone else's house.

'What's wrong with killing whales? Norwegians have always killed whales.' His voice became loud, more insistent. 'Norwegians would!'

'Well, you have your beliefs, we have ours,' was my feeble reply.

By now he was shouting. 'It is our right to kill whales!' he thundered. 'What right have New Zealanders to stop us?' He was working himself into a fury. How the hell had I got into this? How could I escape unharmed? I'm not afraid of a reasoned argument but this was becoming pretty difficult. The children had all stopped talking and were waiting to see what happened next.

Janna saved me. 'It's not right to talk to our guest like that,' she admonished him calmly. 'Now go to bed.' And he did. He just got up and disappeared, without a word. In the morning we woke up late-ish and he was already gone, off to work.

As we drove off to see my own Norwegian friends, fly fishermen I had met at home, I mused again at what a rich and wonderful life my veterinary career had given me.

I'd been to places and met people I would never have met otherwise, and I was the better for it. I think.

The rest of the trip was great. Fishing in Norwegian rivers, meeting Jane in Grenoble and watching her come to grips with her postgraduate engineering work, in French. Finally, I spent a week with Neil in Scotland. We played golf in the mornings and visited whisky distilleries in the afternoon. Not the other way round.

I came home refreshed for a few more years of work. But I never forgot the Norwegian dinner. A strange and funny night where I got in the schtuck without saying anything at all.

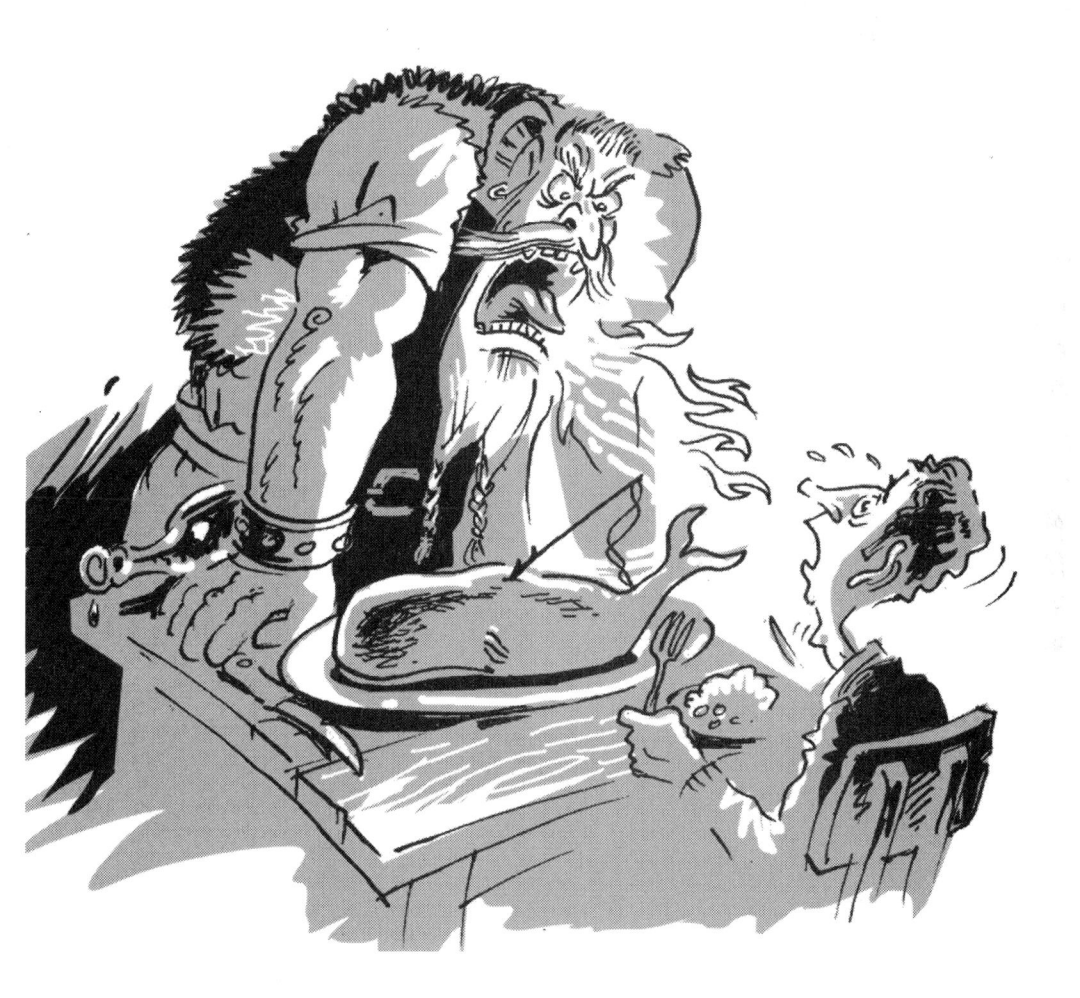

EVOLUTION – PA

When I first started practising in the mid-1970s, vets, especially those in rural areas, had to be reasonably competent in all aspects of veterinary practice. A day might have started off with an early morning unexpected calving followed by looking at a dog and a cat or two back at the clinic. These might have been booked in but quite possibly the owner had just arrived with his or her pet on the off-chance that you might be sitting around looking for something to do. It could be an animal with a skin infection, a broken leg, or vomiting and diarrhoea from some gut infection. And in those days some of the nasty contagious diseases, such as distemper, feline enteritis and a little later on the dog disease parvovirus, occurred on a regular basis. Nowadays these conditions are well controlled by vaccination programmes. Some jobs were simple but others, as they still do, although perhaps less often, tested your skills.

The morning might then finish with a dog spay and a cat castration that had been booked, then the broken leg that had come in if there was time. At 2 p.m. a farmer was expecting you at his property, 60 kilometres away, to pregnancy test 200 cows, and on the way home there could be a colt castration at another property. If you hadn't had time before you left to fix the broken leg then that would be waiting for you back at the clinic. If you were lucky your colleague had returned from his rounds before you and had done that job.

Whatever happened — work was never mundane. There was always the unexpected and you had to be able to switch from being a bovine obstetrician to an epidemiologist sorting out a disease outbreak or growth-rate problem in a mob of hoggets to a small animal radiologist then an anaesthetist and then a surgeon and finally swap between being a cat and a dog specialist and — just to add more variety — perhaps a budgie expert.

With companion animals the diagnoses of any sort of problem was invariably made after a really thorough physical examination and some astute questioning of the owner — although this was not always that helpful! The use of laboratory testing and other ancillary tests, such as radiography, was really only used to confirm or rule out a diagnosis. Routine laboratory testing was not often resorted to as we had no in-house lab and the turnaround time of the Animal Health Laboratory, the nearest being 300 kilometres away at Lincoln, was usually too slow to be really useful. The local hospital, while helpful, did most of the blood analysis but often had difficulty interpreting some of the tests from the different species, and didn't have many of the tests we required for our patients.

So the work in those earlier days was challenging and it was exciting. We were basically James Herriot-type practitioners.

We were generalists and reacted to the situation and dealt with everything the best we could. If there was more than one vet in a practice then as a new graduate you might refer to a more experienced colleague when faced with an unusual situation or when you felt you were out of your depth, but generally you managed on your own. There was little in the way of referrals to other vets because in those days few vets actually specialised in any field. We were jacks of all trades and I was actually quite proud of that fact. While I knew I could handle most situations, I did, after a while, start to appreciate that I was not an expert or really highly competent in any field.

For instance, broken legs in working dogs were common. When I started practising we fixed most of them with plaster casts or by pinning. Pinning involved driving a pin up through one of the broken ends of the bone and out through the head of the bone and the skin at the end of that section, and then lining up the broken ends and pushing the pin back into and down to the end of the other section. It was only effective for some breaks in some bones. Plaster casting was notoriously unrewarding. If the casts got wet they crumbled and collapsed because we only used plaster of Paris. None of that new-fangled lightweight water-resistant synthetic stuff. And if the casts were uncomfortable they would get chewed off. As anyone who has had a limb in a cast knows, these can become uncomfortable and an itch is hard to scratch. Dogs and cats deal with that the only way they know how — by chewing over the itchy area.

So in those early days we became very competent at amputating limbs and there were a lot of three-legged cats and dogs around. It really was the best option for serious breaks when casting or pinning was unlikely to be successful. After all, as someone once said, cats and dogs, especially small dogs, have three legs plus a spare. Having three good legs was a far better option for a cat or dog than three good legs plus a badly mended one that didn't work too well and gave it pain for the rest of its life.

With time, improved bone fixation techniques became available. While I could never claim to be any good at plating bones or using external fixation techniques, Pete J did a number of courses and studied the different processes and became extremely competent in this field. Three-legged dogs eventually became a bit of a rarity in the area.

In the 1980s the country was buzzing and farming was on a high. Not only farmers but small lifestyle-block holders, many of whom were professionals, wanted to join in the farming boom. Diversify was the message and a number of good sheep and cattle farmers came unstuck by not doing better what they were good at, but rather trying new ventures. We suddenly had to deal with a whole new range of animals, all with their own specific issues: deer, goats, alpacas and llamas, ostriches and emus, fitches and even rabbits and possums.

This was a really exciting period for the profession. The demand for high-quality founder animals was there and we were not going to miss out. We learned artificial insemination and embryo transfer, supplying this service to local and not so local beef, sheep, goat and deer farmers. You can read all about these times in 'Angora Anguish' (page 47), 'Helping the Ram Out' (page 169) and 'The Lord God Made Them All' (page 105).

So with time the profession in rural areas has evolved from one where each vet had a go at doing everything to one where many individuals provide specialist services. This has been helped by the trend away from one or two vets in each practice, where you tended to be working alone much of the time and had to be able to handle all situations, to multi-vet practices.

We all have different skills and abilities and interests so in multi-vet practices these days any particular animal health issue tends to go to the person best qualified for the job. Many practices now limit themselves almost solely to one species, for example a large animal (LA) practice might provide an equine or a dairy cow service and within that practice individuals might focus all their work on one area such as surgery or reproduction or mastitis control. A better, more complete service is available to the public when there are vets around who concentrate on a narrow field or specialise.

Specialisation is very useful as one ages, especially in the LA field. A lot of the work in this field is physically demanding so there are not too many rural vets in their mid- to late sixties still actively doing routine hands-on LA jobs. Many have had to quit because they have found a lot of the work has become too much for an ageing worn-out body. If they have not developed a reputation for a specialist skill, with possible referral work from other practices, then they will retire, very often away from the area where they might have spent all their working days. Sadly, with them goes a huge amount of local knowledge specific to the area.

Specialisation has become more and more important and probably essential for the sustainability of rural veterinary practices. In the past the sale of animal health products always subsidised income because in many of these rural practices, particularly the more remote ones, the fees charged are insufficient to cover costs. Too much time is taken up driving to jobs and in non-revenue-generating activities in the clinic, as well as discussing issues and giving free advice over the telephone. Now the animal health remedy market is being seriously challenged by trading conglomerates and certain fertiliser companies that are able to pass on these products at minimum cost to themselves, giving no or at most token animal health advice.

The trend over the years has also been for non-veterinarians to do some of the more lucrative LA work. While these people cannot provide the total service veterinarians can, there are definitely some jobs such as TB testing and pregnancy scanning that they can do. As a result we have seen some jobs, especially the routine and more lucrative ones, slipping to cheaper operators who come into farming areas for a couple of months, take a good deal of the work, and then at the end of the season disappear back to their own farms or other jobs. Some progressive rural practices do now, however, employ LA technicians for this work. This trend will probably continue, as it should, because it then frees up the vet to spend more time doing real veterinary investigative work, sorting out flock and herd performance issues and charging properly for it.

Pete J and I decided to take on different responsibilities and roles in our practice in the late 1980s. It amazed me how quickly I started losing my small animal diagnostic skills and forgot the treatment regimes required for specific conditions when the only small animal work I did was after hours or during the weekends. Various little incidents reminded me that it was time to drop small animal work altogether.

We now have to accept that the romantic days of the generalist veterinarian, the James Herriots of this world, are numbered. 'Progress' determines that we become specialists. For the production animal veterinarian that means providing a service to farmers that helps them determine their opportunities, gives their business direction, and is able to measure and demonstrate improvements in farm performance, productivity and profitability. I believe that the very survival of farm vets depends on us continuing to develop our skills and expertise in this area.

For my part I have always had a strong interest in whole flock and herd production and management and over the years became more and more involved in advisory work. Nowadays it is practically all I do.

This farm consultancy and advisory work has allowed me to continue working long after age and wear and tear would have shut me out of LA clinical work and I would probably have retired from the profession. I'm not ready for that yet.

I love the job and the people I work with and the clients I work for.

SEEN YOURS SENIORS — PJ

In the mid-1980s Ally and I had one of those rare pieces of good fortune that come to some people. We inherited some money.

My mother's sister, our dear Aunt Joan, died suddenly in the street in Wellington, where she was on holiday from her permanent home in Sydney. Joan had married later in life to a widowed man who we saw as rather unfriendly, and pretty damned tight too. He had an adult family, but he and Joan had no children together so when he died the childless Aunt Joan saw our family, her sister's children, as her closest relatives. She would come to visit each of us from time to time, and had a particular liking for Ally and me. She was a bit boring, but demanded little, and was quite lonely, and we always rather liked her visits. She gave me a connection to the mother I'd lost when I was a twelve-year-old, and Ally was her genuine kind self with the old girl, making her feel wanted.

A month or two after Joan's death, and to our real surprise, we five nieces and nephews all received a lawyer's letter, advising that we were the beneficiaries of Joan's will, and we would shortly be receiving a sum of money which, for those days, and in our perpetual state of 'making do' with a growing family, seemed huge.

The result was that Ally and I had our first major overseas trip, and we bought a nice old brick house on three-quarters of an acre in Springlands. It was a significant jump in property for us, and I have been forever grateful to my Aunt Joan for her thoughtfulness.

The house we bought was a very solid single storey, double brick building, with internal brick walls coated with concrete, not just plaster. Hanging pictures was a bit of a mission and involved gearing up with a hammer drill and bits. It was a well-known house, as it had been owned for many years by a loved and respected general practitioner named Brian Bruce. Doctor Bruce was not only a GP, but also served as the local obstetrician and gynaecologist. He had looked after Ally while she was pregnant with Jane, our second child.

The reader may wonder where this story is going, and to what veterinary point, but there is a connection. Mike and Sue Cambridge were farmers in the Waihopai Valley, a hard part of Marlborough's farming country. They became clients of Anderson & Jerram and on several occasions I visited the farm to pregnancy test their cows, or vaccinate the dogs, perhaps to treat a lame bull. Mike was industrious and clever, while Sue has a delightful sense of humour. Like most of the women of that era, she had been a patient of Dr Bruce, who may well have delivered some of her children, but I'm guessing.

What I do know is that Sue had a favourite story about Dr Bruce. He was a regular churchgoer, a solid member of the

Anglican community in the days and of a generation when churches were often full for the Sunday service. Sue always maintained that when Dr Bruce returned to his seat after receiving communion, he would nod in recognition to the many women who were, or had been, his patients. His head would bob up and down for the length of the aisle, and Sue reckoned he was silently saying 'Seen yours, seen yours, seen yours . . .' as he graciously acknowledged his patients. It was a funny story that tickled most people's sense of humour. When I heard it from another friend I was highly amused.

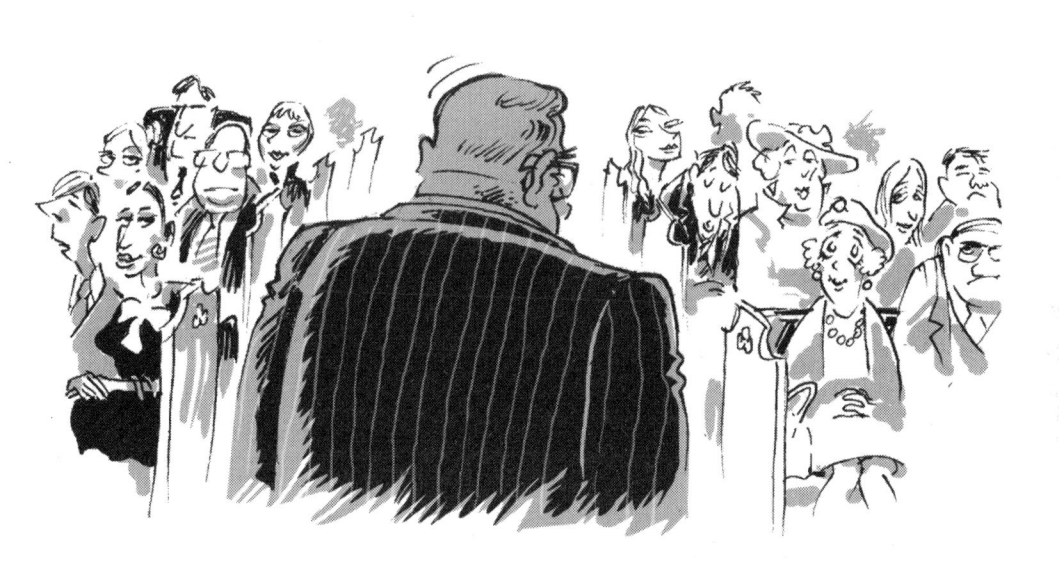

Only a day or so after hearing the story and still chuckling, I got myself in a bit of trouble over it. It was autumn and I returned home one evening from a game of after-work squash to find a message: Would I please ring Mike Cambridge to arrange a visit to pregnancy test the cows. After dinner I rang the Cambridges' number. Sue answered the phone, and cheekily, even stupidly, and on the spur of the moment, I mimicked the slow voice of Dr Bruce.

'Hello, Sue here.'

'Oh, hello Sue, it's Brian Bruce here, and I've seen yours,' I said in a slow deep voice.

There was a stunned silence on the other end of the phone, then in a querulous voice, 'Yes, Dr Bruce, you saw me today. Is there something wrong?'

I was completely bemuddled, and instantly gave in. I confessed it was me, ringing for Mike. Sue was not unfriendly but didn't sound too amused as she passed me over to her husband. Embarrassed at my cheek, I organised the visit with Mike and said goodbye rapidly.

A day or two later I recounted all of the story to a mutual friend, Puddy Sheild.

'Oh my God, Pete,' she said. 'Sue had just found out that day that she had an unexpected pregnancy.' Sue was at an age when she'd thought that was a thing of the past, and it was some years after her previous children had been born. Talk about putting your foot in it.

Sue was very understanding, and we laughed about it afterwards, but I was always just a bit more careful with my telephone calls after that.

Smart bastards don't always get it right.

WRAPPING UP – PA

I am now definitely in the twilight of my career. Looking back I hope I might have inspired one or two young people to train and become veterinarians. It is also quite possible that I have put some off the idea of becoming a vet, and that is not necessarily a bad thing. Throughout my time in practice I have heard young people tell me they are going to be a vet or want to be a vet because they 'love animals'. Well, most people enjoy looking at or being with or working with animals but unfortunately 'loving' them as it happens is not really enough.

A number of those who want to be a vet when they grow up get to the point where they arrange to spend a day in a veterinary clinic to find out about the job, but the sights and smells and general hustle and bustle of surgery as well as the actual treatment animals have to receive is too much and they quickly lose enthusiasm for their dream job. Others might persist with their aim until hormones kick in and social interests alter their direction in life. Or perhaps they are put off by the realisation that training to be a vet takes at least five years of total commitment and hard work at university before they can even start to work. And while they are building up a sizeable student loan their mates are out having a great time as well as earning a living.

But for those young budding veterinarians who enthusiastically pursue their dream, knowing what is ahead of them in the way of hard graft, stress and some deprivations, it will all be worth it. The rewards possible after achieving the veterinary science degree would be matched by few other qualifications. The opportunities it creates are only limited by the imagination. Few other qualifications can give you such a real purpose for living and working.

I have enjoyed immensely my life as a veterinarian, especially as my role has changed from a generalist to a sheep and beef farm advisor. Here our role is more to ensure stock are fed enough of the right stuff at the right time in an environment in which they can happily survive and grow and breed as well as possible. It's more about prevention and welfare and whole herd and flock performance. My work in this area of the profession has been for me more rewarding than if I had worked as a companion animal vet where the emphasis tends to be a little similar to the medical profession — to fix things when they go wrong.

I am helped significantly here by being a StockCARE advisor. StockCARE is a programme to help sheep and beef farmers really find out what is going on in their businesses. It uses comprehensive systems to measure the important drivers of the farm business. The information collected through accurate measuring and recording is used to identify factors that are limiting flock and herd performance. We help the farmer identify opportunities and the most appropriate solutions to improve their business. This programme was developed by one of the most astute practical production animal vets in the country — Chris Mulvaney. I have had the privilege of working alongside him and a handful of other leading sheep and beef vets for the last 15 years.

And would I do it all again? Without doubt, but only if I could ensure I did it with Chick who has been a tower of strength right from my student days through all my working life. She has almost single-handedly brought up our children because during their childhood Pete J and I were just too damn busy working and trying to make ends meet. I hope, though, that I have been a good influence on them and do like to think that because of their upbringing they have grabbed every opportunity that has come their way and given things a go and succeeded and made me very proud.

And, yes, I would do it all again but couldn't imagine doing it without Pete and Ally. Pete is an excellent veterinarian, an inspiring partner and wonderful friend. We have loved the work, been passionate about it, and like to think we've been good at it. My journey through life in Marlborough just would not have been the same without him.

THE FINAL CURTAIN – PJ

It was a wonderful career, rich in experiences of many kinds. We made many friends, and probably a few enemies. Such is life. We have been very lucky to live where we are. It has been great fun.

For the most part I enjoyed being a vet hugely. The great cost was to my family, who didn't see a lot of me for much of my career. I played a fair amount of sport as a distraction from the pressures of a professional life, and that took much of my time too. I would play squash five or six nights a week for an hour, and in the summer I played cricket most weekends. At other times I would go fishing in the mountains, or sailing in the Sounds, although the family could share much of the latter.

Hopefully, my children saw enough of the fun things I did and they felt encouraged to do the same. I think they have done, more or less.

In *Cock and Bull Stories* I spoke of the terrible blow we received at the loss of our beloved elder daughter Jane in the French Alps.

That has certainly taken its toll on Ally and me, and on Tom and Pip as well. Our children are great, personally and in their professional lives, where they're both medical specialists. And I love watching my grandchildren grow up.

Now in my late sixties, I look back on my veterinary career with great fondness, and some pride. We built a good practice, and pushed ourselves well beyond the mundane. Pete A and I remain lifetime friends, and I consider that to be a large factor in the enjoyment of our careers.

Would I do it all again? You bet I would.

My life has continued to develop since retirement. I became a local body councillor, and my work as chair of the Environment Committee, essentially the regional council part of Marlborough's District Council, has been interesting and mostly fulfilling.

I spend a lot of my time endeavouring to ensure that our rivers, streams and seaways remain clean, and our soils remain stable and productive, whether for primary production or long-term conservation. I am deeply concerned at the flawed business and environmental model which is our modern dairy industry. Our rivers and ground waters, and our life-giving soils simply cannot sustain the environmental assault they are being subjected to. Intensification of stocking rates and the massive application of nitrogenous fertilisers is rapidly degrading both of those essential resources.

And there are real animal welfare concerns too, as many dairy vets will acknowledge. The very large herds that have now developed in the South Island as the industry has grown exponentially have been hard to manage for converted sheep farmers, or farmers used to dealing with 150-200 cows. In the smaller herds of the previous era, every cow was known personally to the farmer. Every idiosyncrasy of that cow was understood, and an unwell cow was spotted very quickly. Not now, and I've seen a large herd in Buller where the lame cows were put aside in a paddock near the shed, but not looked at individually. There was no time and insufficient resources to look at individuals. If she came right, she went back in the herd. If she didn't, shoot her. She may have only had a hoof abscess or a stone between her claws, but there was no time to look. And some herds are chronically underfed, as new dairy farmers fail to come to terms with the management of intensive large herd farming.

These problems aren't the norm, but there are enough of them to ring alarm bells.

Our dairy farmers just can't sustain the personal and financial stresses of that intensification and the high debt loads that go with it. It's a destructive cycle, a chicken and egg merry-go-round which has to slow down. The model is not sustainable. Importing massive amounts of palm kernel extract (PKE, a byproduct of the palm oil industry) to feed overstocked cows is another part of the puzzle. It's driven by dollars rather than a long-term view of what's good for the country, and the world. The effects on climate change of removing and burning large areas of tropical rainforest to provide the PKE should beggar belief to thinking agriculturalists.

We farmed mostly sustainably for one-hundred-and-something years, but the script has gone very much askew in the last 30.

I am also concerned about our forestry industry. Harvesting methods have not advanced significantly since the 1970s in terms of protection of the soils, particularly on the steep hill country where most of Marlborough's forests grow. The steep land and schist-based soils of North Marlborough mean precious life-giving topsoil is easily removed and shifted downhill during rainfall in the post-harvest years. I would dearly love to see more thought and investment going into aerial logging techniques. Present systems mostly drag logs along the ground, uphill and downhill, creating bare soil and vertical runnels to channel the soil and water downhill. Cost is the overriding consideration, at the expense of the soils and the waterways. Human safety, a big issue, has improved a lot but protection of the environment is mostly overlooked.

My job on the council has been to try to bring a culture of prevention into our planning regimes. We have to have industry, but we also have to avoid practices which degrade our environment. It is those resource management plans which care for the long-term sustainability of our soils and waters. Developers, and some in primary industry, don't always like the plans, but without them we would still be a Wild West society. I don't believe the farmers I know, and have come to admire, want to see the soils depleted or eroded away, nor the waters diminished and polluted.

These are the issues I have turned my mind to. In these things, I haven't achieved as much as I would like, but I think I've had some small influence on the future of Marlborough.

Will I write more? Yes, but not on our veterinary life. There's plenty to do yet, and other things have captured my interest. The James Cook sestercentennial (that's 250 years since his arrival) in 2019 and 2020 and Cook's times in Queen Charlotte Sound are particular and immediate interests.

I hope you have enjoyed our stories as much as we have enjoyed remembering and sharing them.

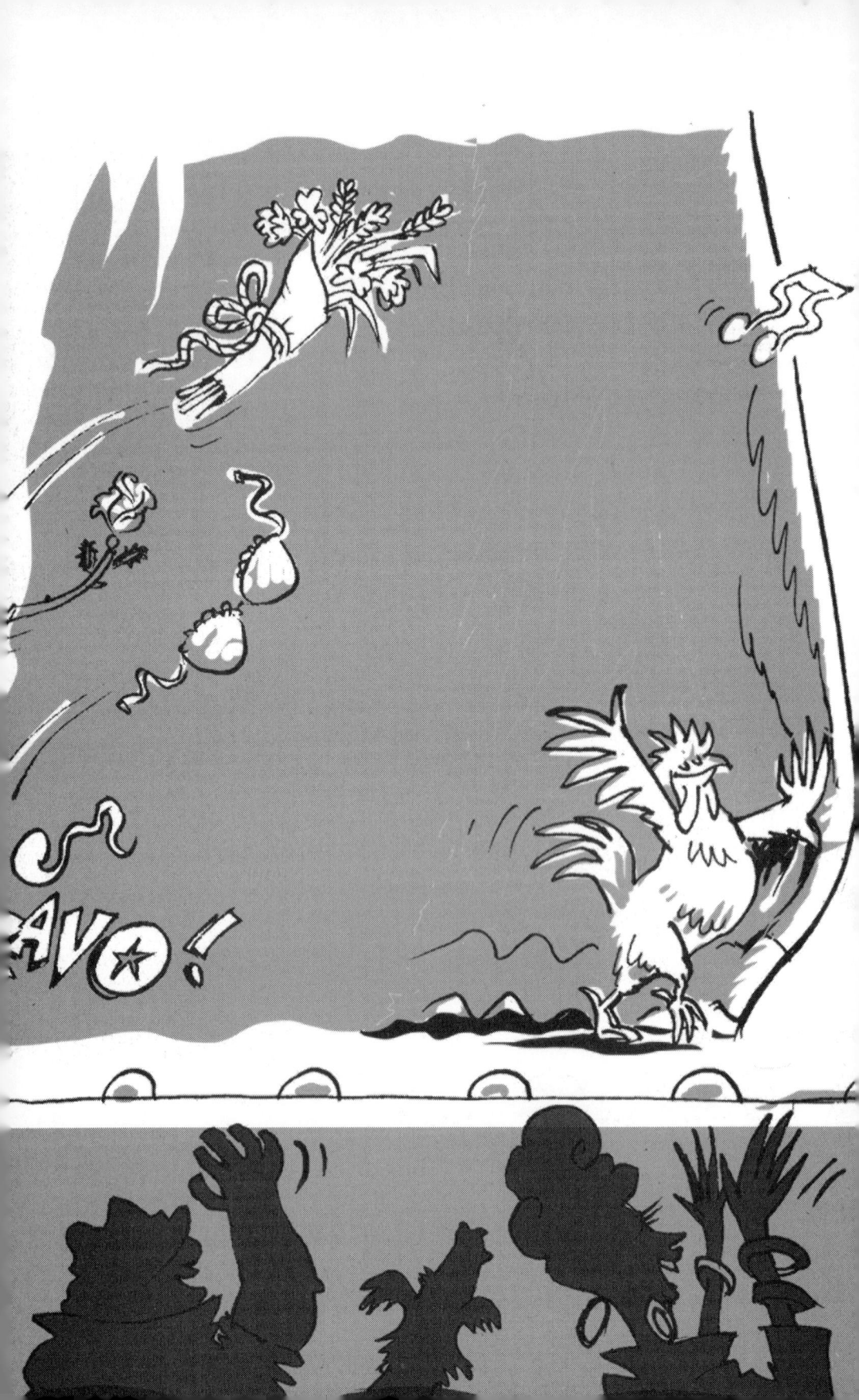

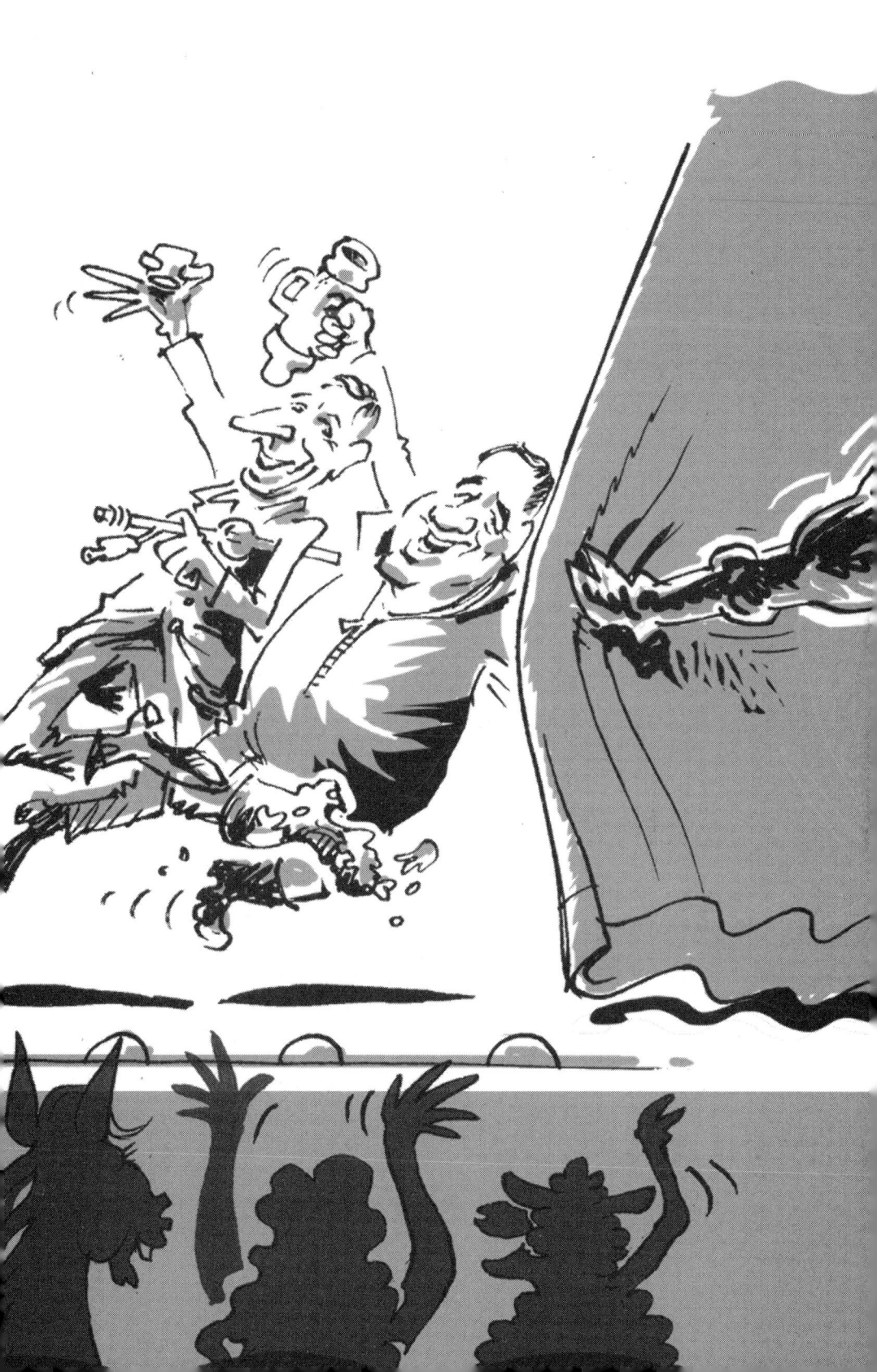

Also available from the same authors:

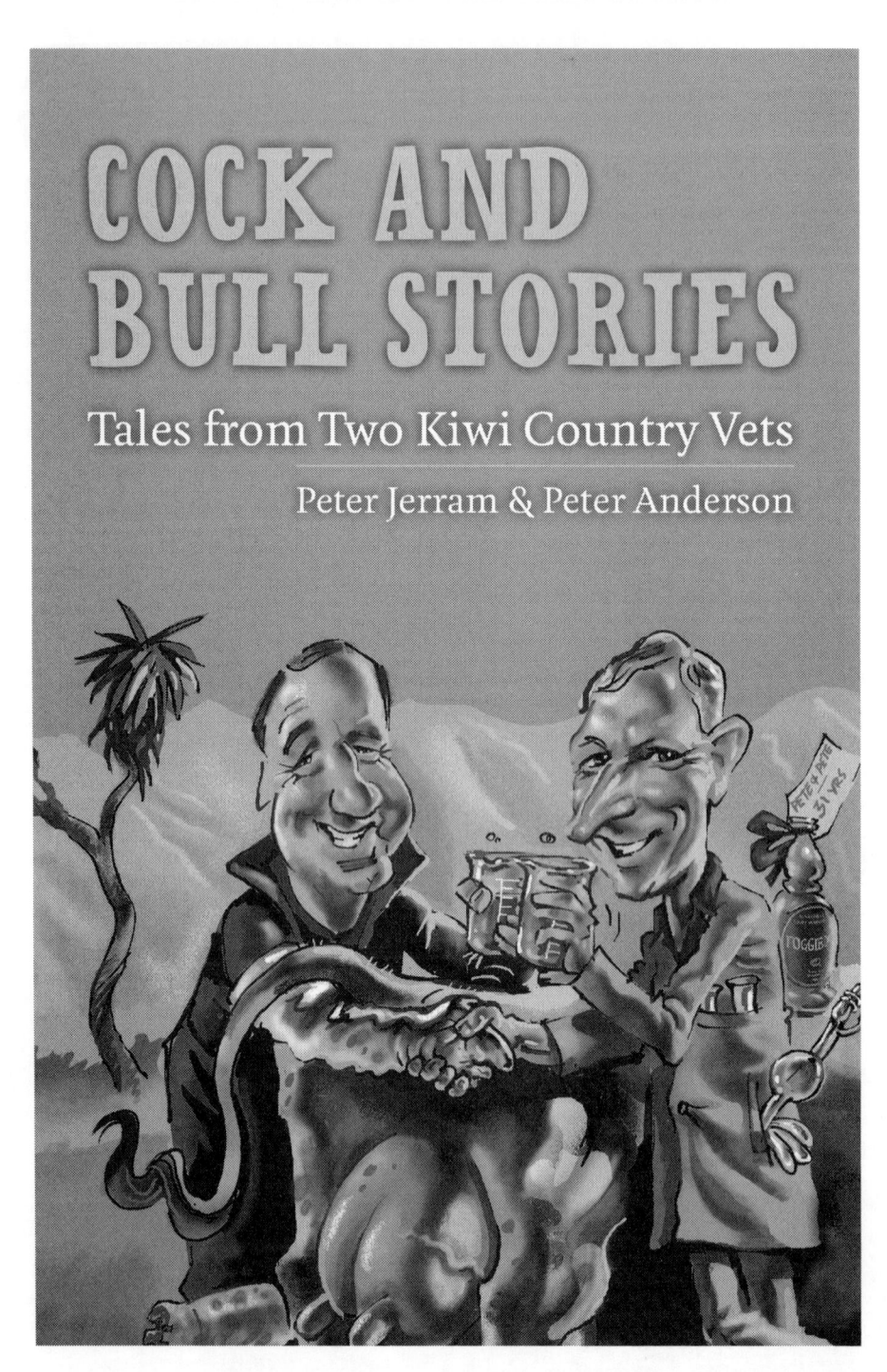

COCK AND BULL STORIES

Tales from Two Kiwi Country Vets

Peter Jerram & Peter Anderson

COCK AND BULL STORIES
Tales from Two Kiwi Country Vets

Peter Jerram & Peter Anderson

Blood testing an elephant. Dodging an angry bull with a prolapsed prepuce. Seeing to 100 stroppy stags. Tranquilising wild cats. For more than 30 years Marlborough vets Peter Jerram (the sailing vet) and Peter Anderson (the flying vet) have been sharing a laugh over cases like these and plenty more besides.

Now, beginning with their first days at work as wet-behind-the-ears young country vets, they've collected their hilarious tales together as *Cock and Bull Stories*.

They've met all sorts of creatures: endearing, dangerous, distressed, angry, comical, heroic, four-legged and two. You'll encounter them in the pages of this book as the two Petes share their insights into country life, reflect on the beauty of the Marlborough landscape, meditate on the nature of friendship and recall their varied veterinary adventures . . . best taken with a therapeutic dram of whisky.

Also available as an eBook

For more information about our other titles visit
www.penguin.co.nz